HOMEOPATHY

FOR

SEXUAL DISORDERS

REPERTORY OF INFERTILITY

PART-1

MALE PART

BY

DR.NIKUNJ TRIVEDI

Dedicated

To

My Beloved Parents

And

My wife Amita
Daughter Arti
Son Parth

Any information given in this book is not intended to be taken as a replacement for medical advice. It is only for reference purpose.
This book provides unique comparative study of the drug picture and disease picture.
Any person with a condition requiring medical attention should consult qualified Homeopath or Medical practitioner.

Order this book online at www.trafford.com
or email orders@trafford.com

Most Trafford titles are also available at major online book retailers.

Printed in Victoria, BC, Canada.

ISBN: 978-1-4251-9113-9

Our mission is to efficiently provide the world's finest, most comprehensive book publishing service, enabling every author to experience success. To find out how to publish your book, your way, and have it available worldwide, visit us online at www.trafford.com

Trafford rev. 2/26/2010

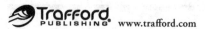 www.trafford.com

North America & international
toll-free: 1 888 232 4444 (USA & Canada)
phone: 250 383 6864 ♦ fax: 812 355 4082

PREFACE:

"What has happened will happen again?

What has been done, still we must do;

Nothing under the Sky is entirely new..."

I read these lines in the book of Gynaecology by Taber, during my final year as an undergraduate. Till date, these lines continue to inspire me, and have led to the creation of my book "Homeopathy for Sexual Disorders". It's my adventure to create different types of clinical approach with Homeopathy.

I am certain that my book will provide students with an 'evidence-based' understanding of the vital concepts. Our great master, Dr. Hahnemann has rightly pointed out that, 'A clear understanding of the basics of Anatomy and Physiology is crucial to restore Abnormal Pathology'. I am convinced that "Homeopathy for Sexual Disorders" (Repertory of Infertility), will offer a sound understanding of the anatomy and physiology of the reproductive systems, and hence be an immensely valuable tool in treating abnormal pathology.

I have tried my level best to use my 28 years of clinical experience, to illustrate many vital symptoms and remedies. The book covers over 75 conditions and provides around 100 remedies. I have liberally taken references from various sources to make the literature scientifically accurate and interesting, which have been acknowledged in the book.

Lastly, I would appreciate honest constructive criticisms and valuable suggestions from my readers to help make future editions more rewarding.

For detailed explanation on Clinical indication and symptom information, I would request you to refer my other book- "Materia Medica Of Sexual Disorders."

CONTENTS Page number

FEMALE PART

UNDERSTANDING THE MALE PART OF INFERTILITY

It is vital to understand the basic anatomy and physiology of male reproductive organs, which comprises of Testes, Epididymis, Seminal Vesicles and Prostate, Prostatic Urethra and Penis, as shown in *Figure 1*.

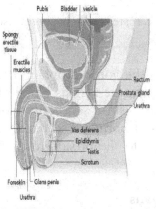

Figure 1 showing the male reproductive system (http://nursingcrib.com/functions-of-the-male-reproductive-organs/)

TESTES

- Two flat oval bodies.
- One on each side.
- Hanging outside the body in a sac called –"Scrotum".
- It is covered tough, compact fibrous capsule called-Tunica Albugenia.
- From Tunica Albugenia, traebecule descend and divide the testes in to a number of pyramidal lobules.
- These lobules are filled up with a convoluted Seminiferous Tubules.
- Each seminiferous tubule is 500mm long.
  Several seminiferous tubules are uniting to form a Straight Tubules.
- Several straight tubules unite to form a Rete Testes.
- These all joins to form a Vasa Efferentia.
- It finally combines to form the duct of Epididymis.

- The whole epididymis having a 6 meters long convoluted tubule which is very long and remaining coiled up together at the back of the testes and ultimately continued as the Vas Deferens.

Function of testes

1. Spermatogenesis:

Spermatogenesis, the process of formation of mature sperm, takes place in seminiferous tubules.

2. Testosterone secretion:

Interstitial cells are the endocrine tissue of the testes, which synthesise the hormone Testosterone.

What is testosterone?

Interstitial cells of Leydig`s are stimulated by the gonadotrophin. The chief products which are secreted in to the spermatic venous blood of adult testes are testosterone and very small quantity of dehydroepiendrosterone. Testosterone (a steroid hormone secreted by the testes), is a male sex hormone. It belongs to the broad group of androgens.

Functions of testosterone (androgen)

1. Growth and development of male sex organs

- Like the seminal vesicles, prostate, epididymis, vas deferens, penis etc.
- Maintenance of the morphologic and functional activity of seminal vesicles.
- Enlargement of seminal vesicles to enable fructose secretion

2. Development of male secondary sex characters

- Development of male pattern of body hair distribution and masculine voice
- Activity and emotional picture of the male
- Increasing the life-span and fertilising power of spermatozoa.

3. Muscular development

- Testosterone has protein anabolic property, thus it aids in increasing the bone matrix and deposition of calcium salts, therefore allowing muscular development
- It also enhances the closure of epiphysis of long bones and thus arrests the growth.

4. Positive nitrogen balance
- It increases the passage of Amino acids insides the cell and improves and maintains the Positive Nitrogen Balance by nitrogen retaining effect.

5. Basal metabolic rate (BMR)
Testosterone increases the BMR. This effect might also be secondary to the protein anabolic property of the hormone.

6. Effect on Red Blood Cells (R.B.C.)
The higher total R.B.C. in males compared to females, is attributed to the effects of testosterone.

7. Effects on water and mineral metabolism
Testosterone causes retention of
- Sodium
- Potassium
- Calcium and
- Phosphate and water also to some extent.

8. Male psycho-sexual behaviour
Testosterone is responsible for development of the male psycho-sexual behavioural pattern.

9. Luteinising hormone (LH) inhibition
Testosterone has an inhibitory effect on LH secretion by the pituitary gland.

Did you know?
Vital Statistics has shown the contribution of
Male (Sperm) Factors are 40% Responsible for Infertility

EPIDIDYMIS

- Has a Pseudo stratified epithelium with tall columnar cells and basal cells.
- The surface cells contain the secretory granules.
- The epididymis acts as a 'store house' of spermatozoa, until ejaculation occurs.
- Even if an ejaculation does not take place, the spermatozoa are produced.
- The un-ejaculated spermatozoa are re-absorbed in Vas Deference.

SEMINAL VESICLE

The vas deference is joined by the duct of the seminal vesicle which is a musculo-glandular sac to form the ejaculatory duct. The ejaculatory duct opens in to prostatic urethra. The secretion of the prostate and seminal vesicles makes up a considerable part of the semen.

The seminal vesicle **does not** store spermatozoa. It acts an 'activator' for the sperms.

The secretion of seminal vesicles contains -
1. Fructose
2. Ascorbic acid
3. Citric acid
4. Inorganic phosphorous
5. Acid soluble phosphorous
6. Electrolytes
7. Protein
8. Ergothioneine
9. Enzymes like Creatine Phospho kinase (CPK)

The secretion of prostate contains -
1. Spermine
2. Citric acid
3. Cholesterol
4. Phospholipids
5. Fibrinolysin
6. Fibrinogenase

All these have important functions for the nourishments of the sperms. The prostate contributes about 20% of total volume of Human Semen.

SEMEN

Semen is an organic fluid that usually contains spermatozoa. It is secreted by the gonads (sexual glands) and other sexual organs of male.

Semen Specific Gravity: 1.028

Semen pH: 7.35 to 7.50

Reaction: Alkaline

Chief constituents of seminal fluid:

1. Fructose:
- It is an index of testicular activity.
- Malnutrition, vitamin deficiency and high fat diet decreases fructose.
- For ejaculated sperms, fructose is the principal source of energy.
- Seminal vesicles are chief site of fructose formation.
- Presence of fructose in semen indicates the patent seminal vesicles.

2. Sorbitol

Sorbitol, also known as glucitol, is a sugar alcohol, which very slowly metabolises in the body. It is a natural production of the body, but it is poorly digested by the body.

3. Spermine

Spermine is secreted by the prostate gland, with rich nitrogenous base. The Barberio test, in forensic medicine bears strong diagnostic value when spermine reacts with Picric acid.

The crystal of spermine phosphate appears when semen is exposed to room temperature.

4. Citrate (Citric Acid)

- Citrate is derived from the prostatic secretion. Its probable role is to help or enhance the sperm motility.
- It helps in semen coagulation and liquefaction, because of citric acid having a calcium binding capacity.
- It helps in activation of prostatic acid phosphatase.
- It helps in promoting hyaluronidase action.
- It helps in maintain the osmotic equilibrium in semen

5. Phosphatase

Acid phosphatase is normally found in male urine in large amount due to admixtures of prostatic secretion.

Action of acid phosphatase allows phosphatic acid to accumulate after ejaculation. After then, it reacts with spermine to form spermine phosphate.

6. Lipids

Lipids in semen are chiefly phospholipids and cholesterol, derived from prostatic secretion. Lipid globules are responsible for the opalescence of the semen. Lipid globules contains macrophages, lipid granules and corpora amylacea, all are from prostate.

7. Protein: fibrinolysin

Seminal plasma contains 3.5 to 5.5 gm of protein like substance per 100 ml. This 'protein-like substance', perhaps fibrinolysin, is responsible for the coagulation of semen.

8. Choline

Choline has a nitrogenous base and is always found in high concentration in the human semen. It is responsible for physiological functions like –

- Lipotrophic Activity
- Stimulation of Phospholipids turn over
- Transmethylation
- Acetyl Choline like activity

Choline is crucial for phospholipids metabolism in male accessory organs and for sperms and sperm motility.

9. Ergothioneine

Like choline, ergothionine also has a nitrogenous base. It acts as a protective substance for sperm and sperm motility against "sulphydryl group- binding substance" and agents. It acts by preventing oxidation of sulphydryl groups, by ensuring fructose utilisation in sperm and enhancing its motility.

10. Hyaluronidase.

It derives from the tubule area of the testes, found in semen with the release of the sperm. It is a mucolytic enzyme.

It depolymerises and hydrolyses the Hyaluronic Acid. It helps and involves in a process of Spermatogenesis. It facilitates the fertilisation by liquefying passage for each sperm through cumulus cells surrounds the ovum.

11. Prostaglandin

Prostaglandin is one of a number of hormone-like substances that participate in a wide range of body functions such as the contraction and relaxation of smooth muscle, the dilation and constriction of blood vessels, control of blood pressure and modulation of inflammation. Prostaglandins are derived from a chemical called arachidonic acid.

12. Other substances

The presence of other substances (as mentioned below) in the seminal fluid is also important.

- Creatine
- Creatinine
- Epinephrine
- Nor-epinephrine
- Inositol

Outlined above is the basic anatomy and physiology of the male reproductive system, understanding of which is important to justify the clinical condition of the patient.

SPERM:

"Sperm is a male reproductive cell, which unites with the ovum in sexual reproduction to produce a new individual."

The sperm is the end product and outcome of a process known as spermatogenesis, which occurs within the testes. The sperm is a highly motile and polarized cell, which delivers the paternal DNA to the egg or follicle, after conception. The mature sperm is 0.05 millimetres long and consists of a head, body and tail. The head is covered by the crown or cap and contains a nucleus of dense genetic material which contains the 23 chromosomes.

Mature sperm are unable to synthesize nucleic acids and proteins.

Spermatogenesis

- Requires 72 to 74 days for germ-cell maturation i.e. Spermatogonia to mature into spermatozoa
- Most efficient genesis at 34^0 centigrade (93.2^0 Fahrenheit)
- Within the seminiferous tubules, cells of sertolli sustain and regulate the sperm maturation.
- Leydig's cells produce Testosterone.

SPERMS & ITS ABNORMALITIES
1. ASPERMIA
Complete absence of sperm, or total absence of seminal fluid or absence of any ejaculates (semen), condition characterised by complete absence of semen.

While "Azoospermia", describes the complete absence of Sperms in seminal Fluid.

Aspermia - The complete lack of seminal fluid and sperms.

- Atrophy Testes:
  - Agnus Castus
  - Ant.Crud
  - Arg.Nit
  - Iodium
- Discharge: Scanty
- Inflammation: Testes
  - Argentums
  - Baptisia
  - Conium
  - Pulsatilla
  - Parotidinum
  - Rhus Tox
- Injury: *Testes*
  - Arnica
  - Hypericum
  - RhusTox
  - Staphysagria
- Indurations: *Testes*
  - Clematis Erecta
  - Parotidinum
  - Rhododendron
- Ejaculation: Absent:
  - Agaricus

Aspermia General Homeopathic Remedies:
  - Agaricus
  - Agnus-Q
  - Ant.Crud
  - Arg.Nit
  - Iodium
  - Rhododendron
  - Sabal Serrulata-Q

2. ASTHENOZOOSPERMIA

Loss or reduction of motility of the spermatozoa frequently associated with infertility.

In Greek – Asthenia means weakness

Sperma means Seed / Semen

Rubrics to consider:

- Atrophy: *Testicles*
    - Capsicum
    - Iodium
    - Kali Iod
    - Testes
    - X-ray
- Induration: *Testicles*
    - Clematis Erecta
    - Parotidinum
    - Rhododendron
- Ejaculation: Without Erection: Sulphur
- Ejaculation : Difficult: Zincum
- Ejaculation: Failing during intercourse:
    - Caladium, Lachesis
    - Eugenia Jambos, Lycopodium
    - Graphitis, Lyssin
    - Psorinum
- Ejaculation: *Incomplete:*
    - Agaricus
    - Camphora
    - Conium
    - Lycopodium

- Ejaculation: Short: Sepia

- Ejaculation: Sudden: China, Phosphrous

- Ejaculation: Thick: Alumina, Medorrhinum

- Ejaculation: Weak: Sepia

3. AZOOSPERMIA

Complete absence of sperm in the ejaculate
Complete absence of sperm, total absence of seminal fluid.
There are two types of Azospermia.
   1. Obstructive
   2. Non obstructive.
To understand the mechanism and process of formation of sperms is called, Spermatogenesis.

Causes of Azospermia
   1. Obstruction i.e. Varicocele, Hydrocele etc
   2. Congenital absence of Vas Deference
   3. Primary Testicular Disorder or Failure

1. Obstruction. –Varicocele,

Varicocele refers to a cystic accumulation of blood in the spermatic cord. It is the most common anatomical abnormality of the veins, especially pampiniform plexus.

Varicocele is mostly found in left sided where spermatic vein empties in the left renal vein. In short, varicocele causes insufficient drainage of the blood from the testes, leading to excessive pooling of the blood resulting into higher intra-scrotal temperature.

Very rarely retrograde ejaculations occur into the urinary bladder in case of -

   • Diabetes mellitus
   • Hodgkin's disease (prior to retro peritoneal dissection)
   • Prostectomy
   • Neurological dysfunction

How to diagnose?
Semen Analysis:
Shows a wide spectrum of information about - Spermatogenesis and steroidogenic function of the testes.

   • Abstinence of 3 to 4 days is very essential
   • Usually 2-3-4 ejaculates should be examined

   • Semen should be obtained by masturbation in a clean sterile glass jar from the laboratory.

- Patient having difficulty in getting samples by masturbation should use silastic condoms, which are free of lubricant and chemical toxins.
- Liquefaction should be at room temperature within 20 to 30 minutes.

Volume (ejaculate): 2 to 6 ml.

Viscosity: within one hour, liquefaction should take place.

<u>Appearance Gross:</u> Opaque or cream coloured

<u>Microscopic</u>

    1 to 3 WBC / HPF

    Ph 7 to 8 (alkaline)

    Motility (at 1-3 hr) more than 50 %

    Sperm count more then 20 million /ml.

    Linear sperm velocity: Clinical correlation of velocity is Unclear.

<u>Morphology:</u>
- Evaluation of sperm structure is important to evaluate the sperm defects.
- Sperm morphology is a stable parameter while motility varies.
- Morphology is less affected by the secretion of various accessory glands.
- Evaluation of "sperm *structure*" is very useful diagnostic factor.

<u>Morphological Properties:</u>

<u>Differentiation of round cells in semen by</u>
- Monoclonal Antibodies
- Semen Culture
- Semen Functional Capacity by SCMPT
  (Standardized sperm-cervical mucus penetration test)

Quick staining method (Diffuick stain) is the ideal for Sperm morphology.

Intrinsic Factors:
- Viral Infection, Typhoid, Mumps
- Orchitis
- Cryptorchism (Relation of one or both of the testes in the abdominal cavity)
- Crypatrchid: A person with un-descended Testis.
- Testicular injury

Extrinsic Factors
- Exposure to Industrial or Environmental Toxins
- Excessive Heat Exposure.
- Acute illness
- Prolonged Fever
- Recreational drug use/ Tobacco
- Alcohol intake
- Drugs:
  1. Anabolic steroids
  2. Exposure to Di-ethyl-Stilbesterol
- Inadequate length of Abstinence Prior to analysis.
- Physical Examination and evaluation of the patient is equally important.

Anatomical Abnormalities
- Decreased Testicular Volume
- Prostatitis
- Hypospadias
- Varicocele

Classification of Male -Infertility Factors
- Genetic
- Neuro-Endocrines
- Testicular
- Uro-genital

Rubrics for Azospermia

Atrophy –*Testes* - Kali. Iod
Atrophy – Sexual Excess After – Staphysagria
Ejaculation absent – Agaricus
Ejaculation difficulty –
- Cimicifuga
- Lachesis
- Lyssinum
- Zincum met.

Enlarged spermatic cord
- Flouric Acid
- Kali. Iod.

Enlarged Testes
- Right. – Arg.nit, Aurum
- Left. – Alumina , Spongia

Erection – Fruitless- Conium, Lycopodium, Platina

Erection –Wanting—Agnus, Calc. Carb, China, Conium, Lyco, Nux.V.

Firmness Increased – *Testes*
- Bromium

Heat – *Testes*
- Belladonna, Nux.V, Pulsatilla, Sabal Ser.

Haematocele
- Arnica, Hamamelis. Ruta, Thiosinaminum

Hydrocele – Left: Digitalis, Rhododendron

Hydrocele caused – Bruise: Arnica

Hydrocele children – Congenital

Cyst – multi-locular   * Apis^{++}

Indurations: Scrotum – Spermatic cord

Testes: Right: Aurum, Conium, Rhododendron
            Left: Bromium, Rhododendron

Chronic:
- Aurum, Baryta Carb, Rhododendron

Gonorrhoea:
- Rhododendron

Indurations: Testes:
- Clematis, Conium, Medorrhinum, Rhododendron

Inflammation

On basis of Cardinal Signs of Inflammation:(***Dolor, Calor, Rubor and Tumour***)

Testes (Orchitis)

Right:
- Clematis,
- Pulsatilla
- Rhododendron

Left:
- Lycopodium
- Iodium

Epididymitis:
- Pulsatilla,
- Rhododendron
- Spongia

Injuries:
- Arnica,
- Calendulla
- Hyperic, Rhus-tox
- Sepia
- Staphisagria

Metastasis: swelling
- Abrotinum
- Carb.Veg
- Pulsatilla

Pain: Testes-Right:
- Arg.Met
- Aurum met
- Rhododendron

Pain: Testes-Left:
- Conium,
- Kalmia
- Lachesis

4. HYPOSPERMATOGENESIS
Oligospermia
Oligozoospermia

Hypo= Low or Less   Genesis = Production

Hypo spermatogenesis is low or insufficient production of the sperm. It is a medical condition affecting the males, resulting in less than 20 million spermatozoa per ml of ejaculate.

Causes:

- Very high fever, Infection, Prolonged illness
- Very High temperature Atmosphere
- Medicines, Drugs, Chemicals
    - e. g. Anti hypertensive
- Tobacco (Smoking, Chewing, Brushing, Snuffing)
- Alcohol and recreational drugs
- Varicocele, Hydrocele, Testicular injury
- Exposure to radiation

5. NON OBSTRUCTIVE AZOSPERMIA

(Testicular Failure)

Fatal derangement in spermatogenesis results in Non-Obstructive Azospermia or Testicular Failure.

Causes are either

- "Sertoli Cell only" pattern
- Maturation arrest
- Hypo spermatogenesis

Important:

Anti-mullerian Hormone (Factor AMH), also known as Mullerian Inhibiting substance (Factor MIF) which is a sertoli cell secreted glycoprotein and is responsible for mullerian duct regression in male foetus. AMH is structurally related to Inhibin and is secreted by sertoli cells in males. Its major function is to allow regression of mullerian duct in male foetus.

The concentration of AMH in the blood decreases dramatically during puberty and persists very low during adolescence [Oxford journals; Human Reproduction, Vol: 14, No 8; 2020-2024; Acq 1999]. AMH controls the Leydig cell proliferation and androgenic functions. It may also be related to germinal cell proliferation.

Research has found AMH to be absent from the seminal plasma of obstructive azospermic patients and deferent duct agenesis.

How to differentiate?

Physical Examination:

1. History of Cryptorchidism in some cases is very important.
2. Small sized Testes (< 15 CC)
3. Flat Epididymis on palpation

Investigations:

1. Serum FSH: High
   Testosterone and Oestradiol Levels are _Normal_
2. Testicular Biopsy to rule out _Carcinoma in Situ._
   (Testicular Intra-Tubular Germ Cell Neoplasm)
3. Karyo-typing: to rule out AZF Defect.

Rubrics to select for Azospermia (Testicular Failure)
Agenesis:

Atrophy: *Testes*

- Agaricus Musc.
- Agnus castuc
- Iodium
- Rhododendron
- Sabal Ser

Induration: *Hard Testes:*
- Agnus
- Aurum Met
- Baryta Carb
- Belladonna
- Conium
- Iodium
- Rhododendron

Inflammation-Metastatic:
- Pulsatilla
- Staphysagria

Retraction:
- Aurum Met
- Clematis
- Oleander
- Rhododendron

6. OBSTRUCTIVE AZOSPERMIA

Obstructive Azospermia, results due to obstruction in either upper or lower male reproductive tract. Here the size of testes is usually 20 to 25 CC with normal serum FSH (Follicle Stimulating Hormone) levels.

Site of Obstruction:

1. Epididymis.
2. Vas-Deference
3. Ejaculatory Duct

Rare Condition:

Young Syndrome: (CBAVD= Congenital Bilateral Absence of Vas Deference)

Investigations:

1. Physical Examination
2. Semen Analysis
3. Testicular Biopsy
4. USG / Scan: Doppler study
   Trans-rectal USG scans to rule out Ejaculatory duct obstruction
5. Vasography

Main causes:

1. Varicocele

A cystic accumulation of blood in spermatic cord is causing varicose and tortuous veins in scrotum. It is most common anatomical abnormality of the veins; especially pampiniform plexus.

Homeopathic Remedies for Varicocele

- Aesculus
- Calc.carb$^+$
- Collinsonia$^+$
- Hamamelis$^+$
- Lachesis^{++}
- Lycopodium^{++}
- Pulsatilla^{++}
- Podophyllum^{++}
- Nux.Vom^{++}

2. Hydrocele.

Effusion of Fluid in to the Tunica Vaginalis of Testes

- Apis$^+$
- Bryonia$^+$
- Iodium$^+$
- Graphitis$^+$
- Pulsatilla$^+$
- Rhododendron$^+$
- Silicea$^+$
- Calc. Carb^{++}
- Digitalis^{++}
- Natrum Mur^{++}
- Rhododendron^{++}
- Selenium^{++}

7. VARICOCELE

A cystic accumulation of blood in spermatic cord is causing varicose and tortuous veins in scrotum. It is most common anatomical abnormality of the veins; especially pampiniform plexus.

Varicoele is most commonly found in the left side where spermatic vein empties in the left renal vein. In short, varicoele causes insufficient drainage of the blood from the testes which cause excessive pooling of the blood resulting into high intra – scrotal temperature.

\#

Rubrics to select:

1. Pain: scrotum
2. Swelling: scrotum
3. Varicocele
4. Scrotum: Skin: colour: Blue
5. Swelling: scrotum: after straining

Homeopathic Remedies:

- Aesculus-Q^{+++}
- Belladonna-Q^{+++}
- Calc. Carb^{+++}
- Hamamelis^{+++}
- Ruta^{+++}
- Pulsatilla-Q^{+++}
- Calc.Carb^{++}
- Lycopodium^{++}
- Silicea^{++}

7. NECROSPERMIA (Dead sperms)

A condition in which there are dead or immobile (inactive) spermatozoa in the semen. In Necrospermia, sperms are produced and found in the semen but are not alive and are unable to fertilise eggs. Over 40% dead sperms in the semen indicate Necrospermia

Causes of Necrospermia

1. Typhoid Fever
2. Mumps, Measles, Chicken Pox
3. STD=Sexually Transmitted Diseases
4. Hernia, Hydrocele, Varicocele
5. Underdevelopment of testes
6. Un descended Testes, Injury to testes,
7. Tuberculoses, Hépatites, HIV, Cancer etc.
8. Genetic.

Rubrics to select

1. Discharge: Offensive:
   Pus
2. Atrophy: Testes:
   - Agnus Castus
   - Ant.Crud,
   - Arg.Nit
   - Iodium
   - Kali Iod
   - Hypericum
   - Ruta
3. Injury
   - Arnica, Hypericum, Ruta
4. Testes: Swelling
   - Apis
   - Belladonna
   - Baptisia
   - Clematis
   - Iodium
   - Pulsatilla

5. Testes: Inflammation.
               Due to Typhoid:
               ▪ Baptisia

               Due to Mumps:

               ▪ Parotidinum
               ▪ Pulsatilla

6. Discharge: offensive:
               ▪ Syphillinum
               ▪ Nit.acid

9. PYOSPERMIA

Pyospermia refers to the presence of white blood cells (WBC) or Pus in semen.Pyospermia is an abnormal condition in which high concentration of WBC are found in human ejaculates during infertility investigations.

Underlying causes:

Infection: with Micro-organisms like

- Chlamydia
- Gardnerella
- Inflammation
- Immunity (Auto-Immunity)

Factors responsible for pyospermia -

- Prolonged Abstinence
- Defective sperms
- Varicocele
- Chronic Prostatitis
- Tobacco- smoking, chewing, snuffing, brushing
- Recreational Drugs--marijuana
- Alcohol
- Fertility drug- Clomiphene Citrate
- Exposure to irritants
- Use of Vaginal Lubricant
- Surgical Corrections like ...
  - a. Urethroplasty
  - b. Vasovasostomy etc.

Rubrics to select:

Male: genitalia: sex:

Ejaculation: Burning—Apis, Bell, Baptisia, Cantharis

Ejaculation: Lemon coloured—Hura Brasil.

Ejaculation: Lumpy—Calc.Carb, Syphillinum

Ejaculation: Painful-Agaricus, Apis, Calc.Carb, Conium, Kreosotum, Sulphur

Ejaculation: Odour Offensive: Flouric.acid, Iodium, Nat.mur, Sulphur

Gleet:
- Agnus,
- Natrum Mur,
- Sepia,
- Sulphur

Urethra:
Discharge
Urethra: Discharge: *Gonorrhoeal*
- Agnus Castus
- Cantharis
- Medorrhinum.
- Sepia,
- Sulphur

10. ERECTILE DYSFUNCTION (ED)

Erectile dysfunction refers to the inability to achieve orgasm with adequate stimulation resulting in either delayed ejaculation or no ejaculation. ED is however different to impotence.

Impotence:

The Latin term *impotentia coeundi* describes simple inability to insert the penis into the vagina. Mostly such condition is due to psychological causes. It is a sexual dysfunction in male that involves an inability to achieve or maintain an erection, sufficient to perform sexual intercourse. The cause may be physiological or psychological: among the most common causes are anxiety, stress and emotional conflicts.

Causes of ED:

Physical:

1. Neurogenic: Neuropathy due to Diabetes
2. Spinal cord Injury
3. Pelvic Injury or Trauma
4. Surgery or Radiation: Prostate or Bladder surgery or Radiation for Cancer treatment
5. Cavernosal Cause-i.e. Pyronie Disease.
6. Hormonal Imbalance
7. Circulation or Arterial Disorders-Peripheral vascular disease.
8. Cardio Vascular Causes: Hypertension

Psychological Causes:

1. Psychological Conditions like Nervousness, Panic Disorders, Apprehension and Anticipation etc.
2. Anxiety Neurosis or Disorders.
3. Iatrogenic
   a. Anti-Hypertensive Treatment
   b. SSRI (Selective serotonin reuptake inhibitors)
   c. Post Surgical or Reconstructive Surgery
4. Age: with the advancement of age, it usually takes place.
5. Use of recreational drugs, tobacco, smoking etc. causing arterial narrowing and vaso-spasm

All these factors are predisposing causes for the Fertility in both sexes; hence it leads to sexual dysfunction.

Classification of dysfunction:

(Root cause is **Psora**)

1. Life long: The dysfunction has always been present.
2. Acquired: At some point, person is able to function without dysfunction.
3. Situational or Conditional: The dysfunction occurs in some situations or in certain conditions and not others.
4. Generalised: The dysfunction occurs regardless of the situation.

After understanding the above stated causes, now we apply the knowledge of Homeopathy to the disease condition of the patients.

Role of Homeopathy

Homeopathy is entirely different in approach from most medical care system based upon a law of similar in a healthy person will cure the same set of symptoms. In every case, Homeopath looks at everything that is going on in the patient's life based upon a "totality of symptoms", Homeopath is covering all the aspect of positive, negative, emotional, sentimental and latent (suppressed) sides of personality.

Usually, I begin with administering Nux Vomica, to most of my patients, to over come the Bad-effects of Coffee, Tobacco, Alcoholic stimulant, highly spiced or seasoned food, over-eating, long continued mental over exertion, stress and sedentary life style, loss of sleep etc. which has become a part of modern hurried and worried life.

According to Boericke:

Mild: Very Irritable, Sensitive to all impression, ugly malicious, cannot bare or tolerate noises, odours, light etc.

According to Nash:

For very particular careful, zealous person, inclined to get excited and angry or of a spiteful, malicious disposition.

On over all analysis, all our great Homeopaths have clearly drawn the picture of present personal condition of azospermic and oligospermi patients in their observations.

To rule the conditions like Azospermia, Oligospermia, the following medicines must be thought of -

Remedies useful for the sperm-related conditions:

1. <u>Agnus Castus</u>: By relieving mental depression, it corrects the desire and improves the functional impotence
2. <u>Anacardium Orientalis</u>: Dual personality, Lack of self confidence with severe depression associated with impaired memory.
3. <u>Argentum Nitricum</u>: Very Apprehensive from the first night of marriage, fearful and nervous, leading to pre mature ejaculations."Erection fails when coition attempted".
4. <u>Caladium</u>: Excellent for smokers & Tobacco chewers. increases the sperm count rapidly in smokers and Tobacco Chewers-Eaters.
5. <u>Conium Mac</u>: Testicular injury Hydrocele, Varicocele, orchitis effects of suppressed sexual appetite.
6. <u>Dioscoria</u>: Suits very well to Tea - Drinkers.
7. <u>Phosphoric Acid</u>: Excellently giving results in Oligo-asthenospermia.
8. It increases the motility of sperms. It increases the Acrosomal activity of the Sperm (Motility).
9. <u>Titanium</u>: Too early ejaculation
10. <u>Tribulus Terrestris</u>: A very good medicine for patient at mid 40's having a partial impotence caused by overindulgence of advancing age.
11. <u>Lycopodium</u>: Proved its great value in sexual dysfunction. (Acquired and situational).Very effective in *premature ejaculations*!
12. <u>Tinospora Cardifolia(2X)</u>: This medicine proves its great value in Anti-Sperm Anti Body positive cases.
13. <u>Orchitinum</u>: Azoospermia
14. <u>Mangifera</u>: Varicocele
15. <u>Potas Xanthae</u>: Impotence

The above stated provides a quick tour of the male infertility therapeutics.

However, it should be appreciated that above mentioned well selected constitutional remedy is an answer to male infertility only.

GENERAL SEXUAL DISORDES IN MALES

11. ABSCESS

An abscess is an abnormal collection of pus which has accumulated in a cavity formed by the tissue due to an infection. It is a defence mechanism for the further spread of infectious material and micro-organisms to other part of body.

- General Remedies:
    - Belladonna
    - Calendulla
    - Gunpowder
    - Merc. Sol
    - Nat. Mur
    - Sillicea
    - Sepia
    - Sulphur
- Abscess on Scrotum
    - Sulphur
- Abscess on Penis
    - Belladonna
    - Baptisia
    - Bovista
    - Sillicea
- Abscess on Testes
    - Capsicum
    - Silicea

12. ADENOSIS

Adenosis is disease of a gland, characterised by the abnormal formation or enlargement of the glandular tissue, either with proliferation, sclerosis, degeneration or fibrosis.

- **General Remedies:**
    - Belladonna
    - Cal. Flour
    - Thiosinaminum
    - Merc.Sol
    - Causticum
    - Iodium

- **Prostate Adenosis**
    - Berb. Vulg
    - Conium
    - Calc Flour
    - Lycopodium
    - Sabal Serrulata
    - Thuja

13. ADHESION

Adhesions are usually called internal scar, band or strand like fibrous tissue which forms an abnormal fibrosis between tissue and organ inside the body.

- Adhesions of testes to scrotum
    - Thiosinaminum
    - Tarantula
- Adhesions followed by injury to testes
    - Arnica
    - Belladonna
    - Capsicum
    - Iodium
    - Conium Mac
    - Rhododendron
- Adhesion – as an outcome of surgery or followed by surgery
    - Arnica
    - Hypericum
    - Staphysagria
    - Thiosinaminum

14. AGGLUTINATION

Agglutination is the clumping of particles in body fluid. The word agglutination comes from the Latin word "Agglutinare" means to "glue together". Usually agglutination found with the following conditions –

Agglutination of semen or "Sperm clumps."

Agglutination means an accumulation and sticking or clumping together of live sperm cell in the ejaculate.

'Head to head' agglutination of sperm occurs very frequently.

It is due to the existence of an electrical charge with sperm membrane leading to clumping.

Two types of Agglutinations found

1. Immunological
2. Chemical/ thermal

    1. Immunological: The sperm membrane acts as an antigen and antibodies are formed against it resulting in clumping.

2. Thermal changes: followed by fever, Heat, Stress.

Presence of metallic spermicidal ions like Magnesium, Calcium, Heavy metals, Chemicals etc.Organic spermicidal substance when contaminate with urine causing interaction with electrolytes and it changes the osmolarity. Bacterial contamination with semen like Escheria coli, Candida Albicantis, E. Histolytica, Trichomonas, Giardiasis.

Rubrics to select:
Semen Discharge
Ejaculation Sticky

- Calcarea Carb
- Staphysagria

Ejaculation Thick →

- Alumina
- Bryonia
- Borax

Ejaculation with threads

- Medorrhinum
- Thiosinaminum
- Tuberculinum

Agglutination - Anti-Sperm Antibodies

Modified rubric: **for (Anti sperm- antibodies)**
- Syphillinum
- Tuberculinum
- Calcarea carb.
- Calc. Flour

General agglutination –

Raised blood coagulability
- Calc. Carb.

Boericke has described, for   Calcarea Carb. Patient,

A person who grow fat, are
- Large-bellied, with large head,
- Pale skin, chalky look,
- The so-called leuco-phlegmatic temperament;
- Affections caused by working in water.
- Great sensitiveness to cold; partial sweat

15. CONGENITAL ADRENAL HYPERPLASIA (CAH)

CAH refers to a group of inherited adrenal gland disorders. They are a group of autosomal recessive disorders of cortisol biosynthesis. Deficiency of 21- hydroxylase leads to excessive production of androgen. It is a congenital condition characterised by elevated androgen which suppresses pituitary gland and interferes with spermatogenesis or ovulation.

Symptoms in Boys

- Early development of masculine characteristics
- Well developed musculature
- Enlarged penis
- Small testes
- Early appearance of pubic hair and hair in the axillae.

Homeopathic Remedies:

The following Homeopathic Remedies to be thought while considering the clinical picture of the disease.

- Pituitarinum
- Testes
- Adrenalin

16. CRYPTORCHIDISM

Cryptorchidism is also called undescended testes or Abdominal Testes.
Means hidden or obscure testis and generally refers to the undescended or mal-descended testis.

Cryptorchidism may be failure of one or both the testes to descend into the scrotum.

The testes first develop within the abdomen, before birth and then normally descend into the scrotum.

In Greek Kryptos = Hidden, secret or covered.
In Greek Orchi = Referring to testicles

Rubrics to select:

In to the abdomen
- Aurum Metallicum
- Iodium

In to the Inguinal canal
- Plumbum met

Retraction Testis
  Right →
- Clematis Erecta
- Plusatilla

  Left →
- Cal. Carb
- Thuja
- Rhododendron

Painful retraction → Agaricus Musc

Retraction while walking → Rhododendron

17. CUSHING'S SYNDROME

Synonym: Hyper cortisolism or Hyper adrenocorticism

It is a rare endocrine disorder caused by chronic exposure of the body's tissue to excess level of cortisol, a hormone naturally produced by adrenal gland. Patient develops hypertension and shows signs of water retention.

A concurrent elevation of adrenal androgen suppresses the pituitary hormones LH and FSH, resulting in low sperm production or ovulation problems. Females may develop male secondary sex characteristics, including abnormal hair growth.

Symptoms

- Obesity especially on upper body
- Moon face – rounded face, Oedema
- Lean and thin arms and legs
- Slow growth rate
- Anxiety and Depression
- Severe fatigue, Irritability, Anger
- Hypertension

Rubrics to select:

1. Obesity
2. Face -Swollen
3. Upper part Body Fat- Lower Thin

Before selecting any rubrics

Clinical Investigations are very important….like

     1. Serum Testosterone
     2. Radiological Scan of Adrenal Gland

Homoeopathically, the following remedies will match with the clinical picture.

1. Calc. Carb.
2. Adrenaline
3. Baryta Carb
4. Cortisone
5. Testosterone

18. EPIDIDYMITIS

Epididymitis refers to an inflammation or infection of the epididymis, a convoluted duct or tubules that lies to the posterior of the testicle. The most common intra-scrotal inflammation is epididymitis.

Patho-physiological causes:

Infection occurs due to retrograde extension of pathogens from Vas deference,

- E.Coli
- Mycoplasma pneumonia
- Entero-viruses, Adenoviruses
- Tuberculosis
- Brucellosis
- Schistosomiasis
- Sexually transmitted pathogens
- Chlamydia trachomatis
- Neisseria gonorrhoae

Rubrics to select:

Male: Genitalia / Sex

Inflammation Scrotum

- Ars alb^{+++}
- Rhus Tox^{+++}
- Rhus Venenata^{+++}

Spermatic Cord:

- Pulsatilla^{+++}
- Spongia^{+++}

Epididymis

- Belladonna+++
- Plusatilla^{+++}
- Rhododendron^{+++}
- Spongia^{+++}
  - Aurum met^{++}
  - China sulph^{++}
  - Medorrhinum^{++}

- Pain: Spermatic Cord
- Jerking: Spermatic Cord
- Urethra: Discharge: Gonorrhoea
- Swelling: Scrotum
- Painful
- Swelling: Scrotum
- Spermatic Cord

19. GONORRHOEA

Gonorrhoea is caused by 'Neisseria gonorrhoea`, bacteria that can grow and multiply easily in the warm and moist areas of the reproductive tract. It may lead to infertility.

The Neisseria can be passed from one person to another through vaginal, oral or anal sex.

It can also be passed on from a mother to her baby during birth through placental route.

Rubrics to select:

Male: Genitalia / Sex

- Balanitis (Inflammation of Glans Penis)
- Gleet (Chronic Gonorrhoeal Urethritis)
- Urethra: Chordee Painful & downward curved erection, usually in gonorrhoea
    - Cann.sativa
    - Pulsatilla
    - Arg. Nitricum
    - Terebenthina
    - Cann. Indica
    - Merc Sol.
    - Nit Acid
    - Nux Vom
    - Thuja
- Urethra: Discharge: Gleety
    - Agnus Castus
    - Capsicum
    - Kali iodium
    - Sepia
    - Sulphur
    - Thuja
    - Silicea
- Urethra discharge: Gonorrhoeal

20. HYDROCELE

It is an abnormal collection of the serous fluid within the Tunica Vaginalis of the scrotum or along the side of spermatic cord.

The serous fluid gets collected in some part of the Processus Vaginalis, when it fails to close, so it remains in Tunica Vaginalis. This tunnel between the scrotum and the peritoneal cavity allows peritoneal fluid to move in to the space around testis.

Types of Hydrocele:
1. Complete congenital Hydrocele.
2. Funicular Hydrocele
3. Infantile Hydrocele
4. Encysted Hydrocele
5. Bilocular Hydrocele
6. Hydrocele of the Hernial sac

Content of the Hydrocele Fluid:
1. Water
2. Inorganic Salt
3. Albumin
4. Fibrinogen
5. Cholesterol and Tyrosine Crystal: Occasionally.

Complications:
1. Rupture
2. Trauma resulting in Haematocele
3. Infection leading to suppurative Hydrocele
4. Hernia of the Hydrocele Sac
5. Calcification of the Sac Wall
6. Atrophy of the Testis.

Homeopathic Remedies:
- Apis Mel
- Belladonna
- Calc. Carb
- Graphitis
- Iodium
- Pulsatilla
- Rhododendron

21. HYPERGLYCEMIA
Derived from a Greek word
Hyper = too much
Glyc = root meaning – sweet
Emia = suffix meaning – of the blood

Causes:

1. Diabetes Mellitus
2. Non – Diabetic
   - Obesity
   - Eating disorders like--Bulimia Nervosa

1. <u>Diabetes</u>
   - Ars. Brom
   - Bridelia Ferruginea
   - Cocca-Q
   - Helleborus Niger
   - Morinda Lucida
   - Natrum Sulph
       - Opium
       - Phosphorous
       - Uranium Nitricum
2. <u>Non-Diabetic</u>
   Obesity:
       - Calc. Carb
       - Graphitis
       - Fuccus Vulgaris
       - Phytolecca
       - Thyroidinum
Rubric:

Appetite: Diminished:
   - Ginko biloba

22. HYPERTHYROIDISM (Hyper-thyroxineamia)

Hyperthyroidism is a clinical syndrome characterised by an excess of circulating free thyroxin (T4) or free triiodothyronine (T3) or sometimes both.

Cause

- Graves' disease
- Toxic thyroid adenoma
- Toxic Multi nodular goitre

Signs and symptoms

- Hyperactivity—Restlessness, Over activity
- Weight loss often accompanied by ravenous hunger
- HOT patient- Intolerance of Heat.
- Fatigue and weakness
- Irritability, Apathy, Depression
- Polyuria
- Sweating
- Palpitations
- Dyspnoea
- Loss of libido
- Nausea, Vomiting and Diarrhoea
- Tremors
- Chorea—St. Vitus` Dance
- Myopathy

Rubrics to select:

Repertory:

- Ext Throat: Swelling, Thyroid gland
- Ext. Throat : Goitre
- Pulsation: Goitre
- Exophthalmic Goitre

Remedies:

- o Iodium
- o Kali iod
- o Flouric acid
- o Platina
- o Ars.Alb
- o Thyroidinum
- o Conium
- o Thuja

23. HYPOTHYROIDISM

Hpothyroidism is caused by insufficient production of thyroid hormone by the thyroid gland.

Cause

Consumption of fluoride in tap water, sodas, bottled water or mineral water.All bottled and canned drinks contain added water soluble fluorides, so in advanced countries the incidence are higher than under developed country.

Thyroid hormones are essential and 'primary regulators' of the body metabolism.

<u>Precautions</u>

Fluoride binds with iodine and prevents it from entering into thyroid. Iodine supplements may reverse the hypothyroidism.

Homeopathic Treatment

The treatment of Hypothyroidism should be strictly based on the totality of symptoms and constitution. The totality in these cases guides for the miasmatic consideration which in this case generally is Sycotic and the constitution is Hydro-genoid. A remedy base on totality may be able to cure this problem on a long term basis.

Some important medicines for the purpose are as follows:

Remedies:

- Arg nitricum
- Cal. carb
- Lycopodium
- Thyroid
- Thuja
- Nat. Sulph
- Graphites
- Ammon Carb
- Thyrodinum
- Iodium
- Nux Mosc
- Pulsatilla

24. IMPOTENCE

Total inability to sustain or maintain an erection, sufficient for sexual intercourse.

Impotence is a sexual dysfunction characterised by the inability to develop or maintain an erection of the penis for satisfactory intercourse regardless of the capability of ejaculation.

Latin term: *"Impotentia coeundi"* describe simple inability to insert the penis into the vagina.

Rubrics to select:

Ejaculation: failing

Erections: wanting

Sexual desire: wanting
- Agnus Castus
- Caladium
- Damiana
- Onosmodium
- Lycopodium
- Phos. Acid
- Conium
- Selenium
- Yohimbinum

25. ORGASMIC DISORDER - ERECTILE DYSFUNCTION

✓ *Premature Ejaculation*

Premature ejaculation refers to persistent or recurrent ejaculation before, upon or shortly after penetration, i.e. ejaculation occurring before the individual wishes.

✓ *Inhibited Orgasm:*

Inability to achieve orgasm with adequate stimulation resulting in either delayed ejaculation or no ejaculation.

✓ *Impotence:*

The Latin term *impotentia coeundi* describes simple inability to insert the penis into the vagina. mostly, due to psychological causes.

✓ *Sexual Anhedonia:*

Absence of pleasure during orgasm with the presence of erection and ejaculation.

Causes:

Physical:

1. Neurogenic: *Neuropathy due to Diabetes
2. Spinal cord Injury
3. Pelvic Injury or Trauma
4. Surgery or Radiation: Prostate or Bladder surgery or Radiation for Cancer treatment
5. Cavernosal Cause-i.e. Pyronie Disease
6. Hormonal Imbalance
7. Circulation or Arterial Disorders-Peripheral vascular disease.
8. Cardio Vascular Causes: Hypertension

Non-Physical condition:

1. Psychological Condition………
2. Panic Disorders, Apprehension
3. Anxiety Neurosis or Disorders
4. Iatrogenic
5. Anti-Hypertensive Treatment
6. SSRI (Selective serotonin re-uptake inhibitors)
7. AGE: with the advancement of age, it usually takes place.
8. USE of Recreational Drugs, Tobacco, Smoking etc. causing Arterial Narrowing and vaso-spasm

Rubrics to select:

1. Ejaculation: Failing During Intercourse
2. Ejaculation: Unable to ejaculate
3. Incomplete -Erection
4. Erection: Wanting
5. Desire :Wanting
6. Desire: Diminished
7. Coitus: Failing

Homeopathic Remedies:
- Argentum Nitricum^{+++}
- Agnus Castus^{+++}
- Caladium^{+++}
- Damiana^{+++}
- Graphitis^{+++}
- Onosmodium^{+++}
- Potash Xanthae^{+++}
- Lac. Caninum^{+++}
- Lycopodium^{+++}
- Acid Phos^{++}
- Conium^{++}
- Euginea Jambos^{++}
- Selenium^{++}
- Staphysagria^{++}
- Yohimbinum^{++}
- Zincum Metallicum^{++}

26. PAN HYPOPITUITARISM

Complete failure of the function of the pituitary gland.

A rare condition where all pituitary hormones are absent or reduced. The condition may be congenital or acquired through pituitary tumours for example. The pituitary gland regulates the activity of other endocrine glands as well as controlling growth. Other endocrine glands include adrenal, parathyroid, thyroid, pancreas, ovaries and testes.

Symptoms can vary greatly depending on the degree of deficiency of the various hormones.

Symptoms:
- Precocious Puberty= Delayed puberty or Puberty failure
- Short stature –Stunted growth-Dwarfism
- Growth hormone deficiency GH Deficiency
- Gonadotropin deficiency
- Dry skin or waxy skin
- Constipation
- Fatigue , Weakness, Malaise, Brain Fag
- Progressive Weight Gain--Increased weight
- Diabetes insipidus =Polyuria
- Frequency of Urine Increased--Increased urination –Polyuria
- Dehydration
- Increased blood sodium level =Hyperkalamia
- Increased thirst =Polydypsia
- Night-time bed-wetting
- Catches cold easily-Sensitivity to cold –Low Immunity
- Reduced appetite –Anorexia
- Wasting- Weight loss –
- Abdominal pain
- Low blood pressure =Hypotension
- Headache and Visual Disturbances and Hot flashes
- Erectile Dysfunction=Male sexual dysfunction
- Reduced body hair armpit and Pubic Region
- Anaemia= Pallor
- Mood Swing, Disinterested expression –Changeability.
- ✓ **Homeopathic Remedies: Based on constitution.**

27. TORSION OF TESTIS

Twisting of testicle inside scrotum.

Sometime, it turns to Medical Emergency and Homeopath has limitations to treat.

In 'testicular torsion' the spermatic cord that provides the blood supply to a testicle is twisted, thus deprived blood supply resulting into 'Orchalgia'. Prolonged testicular torsion results in the death of the testicle and surrounding tissue. Testicular torsion is sometimes known as the "Winter Syndrome"

Symptoms

- Pain in the testicular region – unilateral scrotal pain
- Swelling
- Discolouration of the scrotum-bluish / brownish
- Nausea (parasympathetic inhibition)
- Vomiting (parasympathetic inhibition)
- Light headedness (Vaso-vagal)
- Testicular lump
- Blood in semen

Rubrics to select:

- Testes--Swelling one sided – Spigelia

- Testes- Swelling-Bluish Red- Arnica, Ars.alb, Hamamelis

- Inflammation: Testes-
    - Arnica[+++]
    - Belladonna[+++]
    - Baptisia[+++]
    - Baryta Carb[+++]
    - Clematis[+++]
    - Pulsatilla [++]
    - Rhododendron[++]
    - Spongia[++]

- Swelling-Spermatic Cord
  - Rt. Side: Clematis Erecta
  - Lt.side: Berberis Vulgaris

- Swelling-after Injury-
  - Arnica
  - Belladonna
  - Variolinum

27. UNDESCENDED TESTICLES (Cryptorchidism)

Un descended testes result when the testicle (or testes) is arrested in its normal path of descent, therefore causing failure of testicle to descend from abdominal cavity into scrotum. The testes first develop within the abdomen before birth and then normally descend into the scrotum. Cryptorchidism is also called un descended testes.

In Greek, Kryptos = Hidden, secret or covered.

In Greek ,Orchi = Referring to testicles

Rubrics to select:
- In to the abdomen
  - Aurum met
  - Iodium
- In to the Inguinal canal :
  - Plumbum met
- Retraction Testes:
  Right →
  - Clematis Erecta
  - Pulsatilla

  Left →
  - Calc. Carb
  - Thuja
  - Rhododendron

- Painful retraction → Agaricus Musc.

- Retraction while walking → Rhododendron.

29. URINARY TRACT INFECTION (UTI)

Symptoms

- Strong and persistent urge to urinate
- Frequency of urine greatly increased.
- Nocturia – Night frequency
- Urethritis – discomfort and pain at urethral meatus
- Dysuria – burning sensation throughout the urethra while urination
- Cystitis – pain in the middle of supra pubic region
- Haematuria – presence of blood / pus in the urine
- Fever with rigors
- Emesis – vomiting
- Fever with rigors
- Abdominal pain – Lower Pelvis.

Homeopathic Treatment:

- Apis Mel
- Berberis Vulg.
- Cantharis
- Equisitum
- Sarsaparilla
- Staphysagria
- Terabenthina.

30. WARTS (Condylomata)

Condyloma – derived from Greek word means Knob.

Condylomata acuminate = Genital warts

Condylomata lata = a white lesion associated with syphilis

Condylomata Acuminata:

Small, pointed papilloma of viral origin usually occurs on the skin or mucus surface of the external genitalia or peri anal region.

Other terms for "Condylomata acuminata" are

- Ano-genital venereal warts
- Genital warts
- Veneral warts
- Verruca accuminata

Causes:

- HPV – Human Papilloma Virus
- Multiple sexual partners
- Unknown partners
- Early onset of sexual activities
- Tobacco
- Nutritional status
- Hormonal causes
- Age
- Stress
- Viral infections such as
  - Influenza
  - HIV
  - Herp

Site:

- Penis
- Vulva
- Urethra
- Vagina
- Cervix and
- Peri- anal region

Homeopathic Remedies: for Warts (Condylomata)

- Anacardim Occ.$^{+++}$
- Cinnabaris^{+++}
- Hepar sulph^{+++}
- Natrum Sulph^{+++}
- Nitric Acid^{+++}
- Sepia^{+++}
- Thuja^{+++}
- Lycopodium^{++}
- Medorrhinum^{++}
- Merc. Sol^{++}
- Phosph.acid^{++}
- Sepia^{++}
- Staphysagria^{++}

End of Part One

HOMEOPATHY

FOR

SEXUAL DISORDERS

REPERTORY OF INFERTILITY

PART - 2

FEMALE PART

UNDERSTANDING FEMALE PART OF INFERTILITY

It is vital to understand the basic anatomy and physiology of female reproductive system, which comprises of

- Uterus
- Fallopian Tubes
- Ovaries and
- Vagina

Female accessory sex organs like vagina, uterus and fallopian tube (shown in *Figure 2*) develops from Mullerian duct.

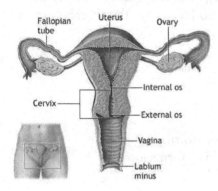

Figure 2 shows the female reproductive system (http://nursingcrib.com/functions-of-the-female-reproductive-organs/)

OVARIES: are pinkish white, ovoid, female reproductive organs. These are homologous to testes in males. They play a prime role in formation of oocytes and production of female sex hormones (like Oestrogen and Progesterone)

Size: 3cm x 1.5cm x 1cm   Shape: Ovoid

Blood Supply: From Ovarian artery which emerges from Aorta, below renal artery.

Venous Drainage: From Pampiniform plexus. Right Vein drains to Inferior vena cava. Left Vein drains to Left Renal Vein

Lymph drainage: Lumbar Lymph nodes Nerve supply: Vaso-motor.

UTERUS

Uterus is a thick walled muscular organ, which is the site of fetal development during gestation. It is consists of three layers –

1. Perimetrium (Outermost layer, loose surrounding tissue)
2. Myometrium (Middle layer, mostly comprised of smooth muscle)
3. Endometrium (Innermost layer)

The endometrium undergoes cyclical changes induced by ovarian hormones at the onset of puberty. If, pregnancy does not occur, each cycle ends with menstrual flow produced by the breakdown and discharge of each layer.

Size:
o Length: 7 to 8 cm, Width: 5 cm, Thickness: 2.5 cm
o Weight: 30 to 40 gm
o Shape: Piriform in shape

It is divided in to two parts:
1. The Body - Upper expanded part forms upper 2/3
2. The Cervix - Lower cylindrical part forms lower 1/3

The body of the Uterus comprises of

- Fundus
- Two surfaces
    - Anterior or Vesical
    - Posterior or Intestinal
- Two Lateral Borders

The cavity of the uterus is a triangular slit between the intestinal and vesical walls. The uterine tubes enter the angles in the fundus.

The apex is continuous with the cervical canal - the junction called the "internal os."

CERVIX

The cervix is cylindrical in shape and is about 2.5 cm long. The canal of cervix is spindle shaped and communicates above with the body of uterus

Blood Supply:

    Arterial Supply:
1. Chiefly by two Uterine Arteries
2. Partly by the Ovarian Arteries.

    Lymph drainage:
- Aortic Nodes
- Superficial Inguinal Nodes
- External Iliac Nodes
- Internal Iliac Nodes
- Sacral Nodes

Nerve supply: Inferior Hypo gastric Nerve

Important:

- Sympathetic nerves T12 and L1 produce uterine contractions and vaso-constrictions.
- Para-sympathetic nerves S2-S3-S4, produces uterine inhibition and vaso-dilatation.

FALLOPIAN TUBES

Fallopian tubes (also known as oviducts) are lined by ciliated epithelium; and lead from ovaries to uterus. Fallopian Tubes are 10 cm long, muscular structure lined with mucus membrane. The main functions of the Fallopian tube include -

- Transportation of Discharged of ovum
- Fertilisation of ovum

Fallopian tube can be sub-divided into 3 parts -

- Infundibulum: It is the lateral end, Funnel Shaped which contains Fimbria.
- Ampulla: It is the medial to the infundibulum which comprises 6-7 cm of the tube on lateral two-third part of the tube.
- Isthmus: It is 2-3 cm long and comprises medial one third of the tube.

Blood Supply:
    Uterine Artery: to medial two third of the tube
    Ovarian Artery: to lateral one third of the tube.
Venous Drainage: Pampiniform Plexus of the ovary and uterine veins.
Lymph Drainage:
- Lateral Aortic Nodes.
- Pre-Aortic Nodes
- Superficial Inguinal Nodes

Nerve Supply:
- Sympathetic Nerves: (T10 to L2) derived from the Hypogastric Plexus.
- Para-sympathetic nerves: derived from the Vagus.

VAGINA

Vagina, meaning "sheath" in Latin, is an elastic muscular canal that extends from the cervix to the vulva. It is a female copulatory organ having a fibro muscular tubular tract leading from the cervix of the uterus to the exterior vulva. Although there is wide anatomical variation, the length of the un-aroused vagina is approximately 6 to 7.5 cm (2.5 to 3 in) across the anterior wall (front), and 9 cm (3.5 in) long across the posterior wall (rear). During sexual arousal the vagina expands in both length and width. Its elasticity allows it to stretch during sexual intercourse and during birth to offspring. The vagina connects the superficial vulva to the cervix of the deep uterus.

Structure:
It comprises of four layers.
- Outer most fibrous Layer
- Muscle Layer
- Sub mucus Layer
- Mucus Membrane.

Function of Vagina:

- Excretory canal for menstrual discharge
- Sexual stimulation and orgasmic response during coition
- Receptive for semen pool
- Secretion of various enzymes helps in liquefaction of semen and capacitation of sperms
- Absorbs the seminal prostaglandins
- Acts as birth canal
- Embryological, female accessory sex organs such as vagina, uterus and fallopian tube develop from Mullerian duct.

UNDERSTANDING *"PHYSIOLOGY OF MENSTRUATION"*

MENSTRUATION

Shedding of the endometrium (i.e. the uterine lining) is known as menstruation. It is a monthly phenomenon in mammalian females of reproductive age. This phenomenon can also be referred to as the weeping of the uterus for the loss of ovum or the funeral of the unfertilised egg

Regular menstruation (26 to 34 days) always accompanied by Pre - Menstrual Molimina, i.e.

- Breast tenderness
- Lower abdomen bloating
- Moodiness
- All are usually ovulatory.(related to ovulation)

Menstrual cycle – Physiology

Cyclic discharge of blood, mucus and certain other substances from the uterus in the reproductive life of a female, at an average interval of 28 days (24 – 32 days) is called Menstruation.

- It occurs every month from Puberty to Menopause.
- Absence: Before Puberty/ During Pregnancy/After Menopause
- Duration: 4 to 6 days
- Composition:
  - Blood (30 – 50 ml)
  - Stripped of Endometrium
  - Mucus
  - Leucocytes
  - An unfertilised ovum

Four phases of endometrial changes
  i.   Post Menstrual Phase (Resting phase)
  ii. Oestrogenic phase (Proliferative phase)
  iii. Progestetional / Luetal / Pre – Menstrual Phase (Secretary Phase)
  iv. Menstrual Phase

Phase	Ovarian Changes	Cause
Resting phase Follicular 1 – 5 days	• Degenerated corpus luteum • Action of progesterone: absent • Slowly maturing follicle • ↑ Oestrogen secretion	• Proliferative changes due to oestrogen from the maturing follicle • Controlled by the FSH – Anterior Pituitary
Proliferative phase 6 – 14 days	• Graffian follicle – maturing • Oestrogen secretion - ↑ • On day 14 – ovulation occurs • Corpus luteum formation begins	• Action of oestrogen continuing • Action of FSH is inhibited by ↑ oestrogen level

Menstrual phase Starts on 28th day 4 – 6 days Blood Mucus Endometrium Unfertilised ovum	• Degradation of corpus luteum (Placental gonadotrophin is important for further growth of corpus luteum, hence in absence of pregnancy, no placental gonadotrophin present)	

FEMALE SEXUAL DISORDERS
1. ABORTION

An abortion is the removal or expulsion of the embryo or foetus from the uterus; resulting in or caused by its death with the arrested progress to grow.

- **Abortion 1st Trimester**
    - Four weeks - 1st Month
        - Apis Mellifica $^{+++}$
        - Caulophylum $^{)++}$
        - Viburnum Opulus $^{++}$
    - Six weeks – One & half month
        - Ipeca
        - Sanguin
        - Spongia
    - Eight weeks-2^{ed} month
        - Kali Carb
        - Cimicifuga
        - Sabina
        - Secal Cor
    - Twelve weeks -3rd month
        - Apis Mel
        - Crocus Sativa
        - Kreosotum
        - Trili. P
        - Eup. Perf
        - Merc. Cor
        - Ustiligo
        - Kali carb
        - Sabina
        - Secalae Cor

- **Abortion 2nd Trimester**
  - Sixteen weeks - 4th Month
    - Apis
    - Caulophyllum
    - Eup.perf
    - Merc Cor
- **Threatened Abortion**
    - Caulophyllum
    - Sepia
  - Twenty weeks - 6th Month
    - Sepia
    - Ars.alb
    - Lac Can
    - Plumbum
    - Ruta
  - Twenty-eighth Weeks -7th Month
    - Ruta
    - Sepia
  - Thirty two Weeks -8th Month
    - Pulsatilla
  - Thirty Six weeks – 9th Month
    - Opium
  - Intra Uterine foetal Death
    - Pulsatilla
    - Ruta
    - Syphillinum
  - Abortion associated with anaemia
    - Sepia
  - Abortion associated with Incompetent Os
    - Caulophyllum
  - Abortion associated with convulsion
    - Absinthium

2.ABSCESS

An abscess is an abnormal collection of Pus which has accumulated in a cavity formed by the tissue due to an infection.

It is a defence mechanism for the further spread of infectious material to other part of body.

General Homeopathy Remedies

- o Belladonna
- o Calendula
- o Gunpowder
- o Merc. Cor
- o Nat. Mur
- o Silicea
- o Sepia,
- o Sulphur

- Abscess-**Rt. Ovary**
  - o Belladonna
  - o Rhus Tox

- Abscess-**Lt. Ovary**
  - o Lachesis

3. ADENOSIS

A disease of a gland, characterised by the abnormal formation or abnormal enlargement of the glandular tissue, accompanied by either proliferation or sclerosis or degeneration or fibrosis.

General Homeopathy Remedies

- o Belladonna
- o Cal. Flour
- o Thiosinaminum
- o Merc. Sol
- o Causticum
- o Iodium

- Breast Adenosis
  - o Baryta Carb
  - o Belladonna
  - o Conium
  - o Calc Flour
  - o Iodium
  - o Lac.can
  - o Phytolecca
  - o Thiosinaminum

4. ADHESION

Adhesions are usually called internal scar, band or strand like fibrous tissue which forms an abnormal fibrosis between tissue and organ inside the body.

Homeopathic Remedies

- Adhesions in the pelvic cavity followed by surgery (Surgical Adhesions)

  o Staphysagria
  o Thiosinaminum
  o Calc Flour

- Followed by Dilatation and Curettage (D & C)

  o Arnica,
  o Belladonna
  o Hypericum
  o Staphysagria

- Adhesion as an outcome of surgery or followed by general surgery
  o Arnica
  o Hypericum
  o Staphysagria
  o Thiosinaminum

5. AGGLUTINATION

Agglutination is the clumping of particles in body fluid, i.e. the act of uniting by other tenacious substances. The word agglutination comes from the Latin word "Agglutinare" means to "glue together". Usually agglutination found with the following conditions.

Homeopathy Remedies

- Leucorrhoea ACRID → (Soreness with Itching)
  - o Alumina
  - o Sepia
  - o Pulsatilla
  - o Nit. Acid
- Leucorrhoea Forming a clot
  - o Bovista
- Leucorrhoea Stains Linen (because of Trichomonas or Giardiasis)
  - o Merc Sol.
  - o Lil. Tig
  - o Nit. Acid
  - Leucorrhoea Yellow
    - o Lac. D
- Leucorrhoea Albuminous
  - o Ammonium .Mur
  - o Borax
  - o Nat. mur
  - o Sepia
- Leucorrhoea Candiaiasis (Moniliasis)
  - o Alumina
  - o Cal. Phos
  - o Mezerum
  - o Platina
  - Leucorrhoea Thick
    - o Alumina
    - o Bryonia
    - o Borax
- General agglutination – Raised blood coagulability
  - o Calc. Carb.
  - o Syphyllinum

6. AMENORRHOEA

Amenorrhoea derived from Greek

✓ A= Negative or Absent
✓ Men= Month
✓ Rhoia= Flow

Amenorrhoea refers to absence of menstruation in a woman of reproductive age. A woman who has never menstruated is said to suffer from Primary amenorrhoea. On the other hand, a woman who has established menstruation, but whose menstruation has ceased for six months is said to suffer from Secondary Amenorrhoea.

Homeopathy Remedies

- Menstruation: Caesation:
    o Graphitis
    o Lachesis
    o Pulsatilla
    o Sanguinaria
    o Asoca Janosia-Q

- Menstruation: Delayed
    o Calc. Carb.
    o Caulophylum
    o Ignatia
    o Pulsatilla
    o Phosphorous
    o Nat. Mur

- Menstruation: Absent: Long Period
    o Weisbeden Aqua
    o Pulsatilla—Q
    o Janocia Asoca-Q

7. ANOVULATION

Anovulation refers to absence of ovulation or failure to ovulate

Factors responsible for Anovulation:

- Stress, new environment

- Chronic mental illness, such as depression

- Chronic physical illness, such as inflammatory bowel disease, poorly controlled diabetes, tuberculosis, or anaemia

- Under nutrition, specific nutrient deficiencies, inadequate body fat
- Prolonged or continuous physical exertion

- Various pharmaceutical (especially phenothiazines) and recreational drugs.

- Hormonal imbalances, such as prolactin or testosterone excess (e.g., polycystic ovary syndrome), hyper- or hypothyroidism, adrenal insufficiency or Cushing's syndrome.

- Pituitary or ovarian failure.

- Prolonged use of birth control pills:

Homeopathic Approach:
  o Apis Mel
  o Conium
  o Iodium
  o Pulsatilla

8. ASHERMAN'S SYNDROME (Gynaetresia)

Asherman's Syndrome is the presence of intra- uterine adhesions that typically occur as a result of scar formation after uterine surgery; especially after a dilation & curettage. The adhesion may lead to amenorrhoea and/or infertility.

Uterine walls adhere to one another; usually caused by uterine inflammations [Dorland: 28th edition]

Occlusion of sore part of the female genital tract; especially of the vagina.

Symptoms

- Amenorrhoea (No menstrual flow) or decreased flow
- Infertility
- Recurrent miscarriages

Rubrics to select

Female: Genitalia: Sex: Os Uteri: stenosis:
   o Conium

Homeopathic Approach

   o Apis^{+++}
   o Ars.alb^{+++}
   o Belladonna^{+++}
   o Lycopodium^{+++}
   o Lachesis^{+++}
   o Pulsatilla^{+++}
   o Sabina^{+++}
   o Thiosinaminum. $^{+++}$
   o Bryonia^{++}
   o Hamamelis. $^{++}$
   o Iodium^{++}
   o Lyssinum^{++}
   o Sepia^{++}
   o Silicea^{++}
   o Sulphur^{++}
   o Veratrum Alb^{++}

9. BACTERIAL VAGINOSIS

Bacterial Vaginosis (BV) is the most common cause of vaginal infection (vaginitis). For grammatical reasons, some people prefer to call it vaginal bacteriosis. It is NOT generally considered to be a sexually transmitted infection (see below). BV is caused by an imbalance of naturally occurring bacterial flora, and should not be confused with yeast infection (candidiasis), or infection with *Trichomonas vaginalis* (trichomoniasis) which are not caused by bacteria.

Rubrics to select:

Leucorrhoea:

1. Leucorrhoea Acrid - Excoriating
     o Ars.alb, Borax, Merc.Cor, Sepia
2. Leucorrhoea Copious
     o Borax, Calc.Carb, Graphitis, Sepia
3. Leucorrhoea Frothy
     o Aethusa, Borax, Trilium
4. Leucorrhoea Forming a Clot
     o Alumina, Borax, Nat.mur
5. Leucorrhoea Gushing
     o Borax, Calc.Carb, Graphitis
6. Leucorrhoea Hot
     o Borax
7. Leucorrhoea Itching
     o Kreosotum-Q
8. Leucorrhoea Jelly like
     o Sabina-Q
9. Leucorrhoea Purulent
     o Fagopyrum, Pulsatilla, Sepia

10. Leucorrhoea Ropy, Stringy, Tenacious :Alumina,Graphitis, Nit.Acid

11. Leucorrhoea Staining Linen : Kreosotum-Q, Lachesis

12. Leucorrhoea Tenacious : Alumina, Graphitis, Nit.Acid

13. Leucorrhoea in Vaginismus : Ignatia

14. Leucorrhoea white
   o   Ovarium, Palladium, Platina
15. Leucorrhoea yellow
   o   Sepia

10.   BLIGHTED OVUM

Blighted Ovum refers to a fertilised egg that develops a placenta and membrane but no embryo.
It is an embryonic gestation which has implanted but not developed.
Pregnancy stopped developing very early & where amniotic sac contains amniotic fluid but no foetal pole.

Rubrics to select:

Female Genitalia: Sex:

Pregnancy: Development: arrested

Pregnancy: Development Cessation

Pregnancy: Development Mole

Homeopathic Remedies:

o Syphillinum^{+++}

o Apis Mel^{++}

o Pulsatilla^{++}

11. CANDIDIASIS

Candidiasis is commonly called yeast infection or thrush. It is a fungal infection of any of the candida species; amongst all *Candida albicans* is the most common.

When it manifest in mouth it is called Oral thrush.

Rubrics to select:

Leucorrhoea

Leucorrhoea Albuminous

       o   Borax, Nat.Mur, Sepia
       o   Ars.alb, Alumina, Cal phos, Platina, Skookum chuk

Leucorrhoea Itching
       o   Cal Carb, Kreos, Sepia

Leucorrhoea Jelly like
       o   Graphitis

Leucorrhoea Smelling like
       o   Causticum, Calendula

Leucorrhoea Milky
       o   Calc, Kali Mur, Puls, Sepia
       o   Borax, Calc phos, Ignatia, Phosph

Leucorrhoea White

       o   Borax, Graphitis Nat Mur, Sepia

       o   Ars alb, Alumina,Calc phos, platina, pulsatilla

12. CERVICAL STENOSIS

Stenosis refers to any passage of the body that is narrower than usual or blocked.

Cervical Stenosis refers to a condition in which the opening of the cervix is narrower than usual or blocked.

Homeopathic Approach

- Adhesion
    - o Bryonia
- General sensation of Adhension of the inner part
    - o Rhus Tox, Thiosi, Plumbum, Sepia, sulphur
- Sensation of a plug
- Constriction
- Contraction
- Chocking
    - o Belladonna
    - o Causticum
    - o Chammmomilla
    - o Lac can
    - o Lycopodium,
    - o Plumbum me
    - o
- Deposit : Caeseous

    - o Calc.Carb
    - o Causticum
    - o Mezerum
- Narrow:
    - o Belladonna

13. CERVICITIES

Cervicities refers to inflammation of the cervix of the uterus.
An inflammation of the cervix; the cervix is a lower end of uterus that opens into the vagina.

Common causes

 Pathological
 Sexual Transmitted Disease
 Gonorrhoea
 Chlamydia
 Herpes

Mechanical:
IUCD, Sensitivity to Latex (Condom)
Spermicide- Tampoons, Sanitary napkins.

Symptoms:

Purulent (pus) discharge, Pelvic pain, Backache,
Urinary Complain, Frequent UTI resulting in Cervicities.

Homeopathic Renedies:

Cervicites:

- o Ars Alb^{+++}
- o Belladonna
- o Merc Cor
- o Lycopodium
- o Argentum nit^{++}
- o Calendula
- o Nit Acid
- o Sepia

14. CHLAMYDIA

Chlamydia trichomatis is a bacterium that can cause sexually transmitted infection, and damages the woman's reproductive organs. Chlamydia infection is very common among young adults and teenagers.

Three species of Chlamydia

- Chlamydia trichomatis
- Chlamydia muridarum
- Chlamydia suis

Chlamydia Infection in female resulting in to

- Cervicities
- Fitz-Hugh-Curtis syndrome
- PID(Pelvic inflammatory Disease)
- Ectopic pregnancy
- Vaginal Bleeding
- Painful Intercourse
- Fever
- Dysuria
- Reactive arthritis(Reiter's Syndrome)

Homeopathic Remedies:

- o Ars Alb^{+++}
- o Belladonna^{+++}
- o Borax^{+++}
- o Merc Cor^{+++}
- o Lycopodium^{+++}
- o Syphillinum^{+++}
- o Arg nit^{++}
- o Calendulla^{++}
- o Medorrhinum^{++}
- o Nit Acid^{++}
- o Sepia^{++}
- o Skukoom Chuck^{++}

15. CHOCOLATE CYST

It is a condition in which the functional endometrial tissue is present outside the uterus. It is often confined to the pelvis, involving the ovary, the ligaments, pouch of Douglas and the utero-vesical peritoneum.

Homeopathic Remedies:

- o Apis Mel.
- o Calcarea Carb
- o Conium
- o Lachesis
- o Thuja
- o Bovista
- o Bufo rana
- o Colocynth
- o Iodium
- o Platina
- o Rhus tox

16. DYSMENORRHOEA

Dysmenorrhoea refers to painful menstruation.

Homeopathic Remedies:

- o Belladonna
- o Cactus
- o Caulophyllum
- o Cimicifuga
- o Erigeron
- o Canadense
- o Millifolium
- o Pulsatilla
- o Ustiligo
- o Veratrum V
- o Cal carb
- o Chammomilla
- o Colocynth
- o Conium
- o Discoria
- o Graphitis
- o Ignatia
- o Lac can
- o Platina
- o Rhustox
- o Sabina
- o Sec cor
- o Sepia
- o Tuberculinum

17. DYSPARUNIA

(Coitalgia) = Painful Intercourse

Vaginismus is an involuntary contraction of muscles around the opening of vagina, which makes sexual intercourse painful or impossible.
It is a condition which affects woman's ability to engage in any form of vaginal penetration or intercourse.

Homeopathic Remedies:

- Cactus$^{+++,}$
- Cimicifuga
- Ignatia
- Pulsatilla
- Plumbum
- Silicea
- Belladonna^{++}
- Berberis Vulgaris
- Cantharis
- Caulophyllum
- Cimicifuga
- Hamamelis
- Murex
- Lycopodium
- Arg.Nit^{++++}
- Lyssin
- Natrum Mur
- Platina
- Sepia
- Staphysagria

18. ENDOMETRIOSIS

Endometriosis refers to the presence of endometrial tissue outside the uterine cavity.

- **Common site**

The spread of endometriosis is confined to the peritoneal or serosal surface of intra-abdominal organs i.e. ovaries, posterior surface of the broad ligament, pouch of Douglass and utero-sacral ligaments.

- **Rare Site**
  - o Serosal surface of large & small intestine.
  - o Urethras & Bladder
  - o Vagina
  - o Any surgical scar
  - o Rarely → plural cavity

- **Age:**

Disease usually starts in the mid 30's with close association with infertility and as a part of manipulative and invasive procedures of infertility investigations.

  - It regresses during pregnancy and menopause

- **Causes: Aetiology:**
  - o Retrograde flow of menstrual blood travels through fallopian tubes is responsible for causing intra-abdominal endometriosis. Its spread to distant sites is responsible either due to lymphatic or circulatory system.
  - o The blood does not have natural way out, so bleeding occurs inside the ovaries in ovarian endometriosis.
  - o Another possible cause is coelomic metaplasia i.e. transformation of coelomic epithelium in to endometrial like glands.
  - o Inherited dyscrasias....like.
    - ❖ Thyroid Crisis
    - ❖ Allergies—Hay Fever, Vasomotor Rhinitis, Asthma
    - ❖ Long history of abdominal and digestion complain with E.H. and yeast infection leading to leucorrhoea.

- **Pathology:**

Pathological Changes.

Hyperplasia of the endometrial tissues and cysts in ovaries adheres to intestine, fallopian tubes and surroundings.

Hyperplasia within the uterus results in to adhesions, blocked fallopian tubes and sometime resulting in to Hydro salpinx

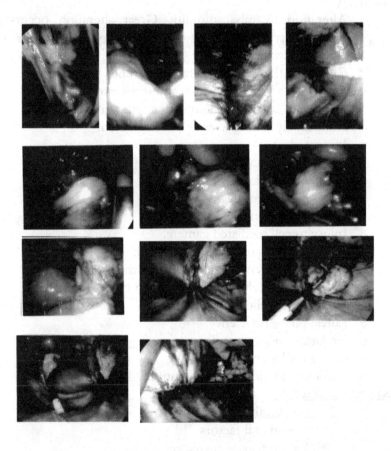

- **Signs & symptoms:**
  - Pelvic pain + Midline pelvic pain
  - Pelvic mass
  - Alteration of menstrual flow
  - Infertility
  - Dysparunia

Complication

  - Alteration in tubal motility. Great alteration occurs in muco-cillary lining of the tube; ciliary movements get affected seriously.
  - Chronic inflammation of fallopian tube.
  - Distortion of fallopian tube and ovarian relation causing impaired follicle transfer through tubes
  - Abnormally raising level of prostaglandin.
  - Increased
    - Prostaglandin
    - Cytokines
    - Macrophages
  - Pelvic Adhesion
  - Injury to cell mediated gamete.
  - Increased presence of auto antibodies
  - Increased presence of anti-endometrial antibodies.
  - Impaired folliculogenesis leading to cyst
  - Un rupture follicle syndrome
  - Luteal phase deficiency
  - Enhanced phagocytosis of sperm
  - Hyper prolectinaemia
  - Difficult nidation or implantation
- **Predisposing factors:**
  - Psychological:
    - Emotional factors
    - Latent fear of sexual act
    - Exploitation

- General:
  - Low Immunity
  - Fertility drugs induced during treatment
  - Over stimulations of the ovaries
- **How to diagnose endometriosis?**
  - Diagnosis made easier by History taking
  - Physical Examination →Pelvic Exam: P/V-P/R

Investigations:
- USG
- Laparoscopy
- Biopsy
- Barium Enema
- I.V.P (Intra venous pyelography)
- I.V. Urogram
- C.T./ Abdominal Scan
- M.R.I.
- Serological Blood Test
  - Serum Markers—C.A.125
  - Anti-endometrial Anti-body test.

- **Aggravation:**

Usually occurs: before, during and after menstruation.
  - Pain gets worse with time and regresses as age advances.
  - It regresses during pregnancy and after menopause.
  - Pain: severe pelvic pain with colic, supra-pubic, mid-pelvic, back, down the thighs
  - Dysparunia (painful intercourse)
  - Dyschasia (pain while defeacation)
  - Dysuria (painful urination)
  - Dyspepsia – Colitis- Irritable bowel syndrome (IBS)
  - Derangement in normal patho-physiology=Adhesions
  - Fibrosis
  - Hydrosalpinx

- **Endometriosis associated with …**
1. Emotional upset.
   - Mood swings, changeable mood, emotional upset, sentimental, loss of interest in life, suppressed emotions come on surface by weeping
2. Pain
   - Dyschaesia - Pain during defecations
   - Dysparunia - Pain during intercourse
   - Dysuria - Pain during urination
3. Periodicity
   - Every four weeks the menstrual cycles are shortened to three weeks
   - Because of weak progesterone level, as there is a poor development of Corpus Luteum called as - Luteal Phase Deficiency.
4. Changeable bleeding and discharge
   Vaginal Bleeding with Discharge - Brown, Black, Bloody, thick-shreds, stringy, Watery Copious, Profuse, Clotted. The consistency, Quantity, and Flow varies with the cyclical changes in Endometrium.

- **Regression:**
Endometriosis regresses during…
   - Pregnancy
   - Lactation and after
   - Menopause

Homeopathic Treatment:
Endometriosis is an osis which means that it is a sycotic.
As endometriosis itself a very complicated condition where approach to treatment is observed under…
1. Miasmatic
2. Constitutional and
3. Pathological aspects.
4. Evaluating Psycho somatic ways

Following Homeopathic Medicines proved its effectiveness.
- Staphysagria (Stavesacre)
  - *(Psycho) --Psychological Symptoms of Staphysagria.*
  - Ill effects of anger and insults resulting in to irritability which reflects on Hormonal Imbalance. (Suppression)
  - Hormonal Imbalance leads to malfunction of the organs.
  - Violent outburst of passions.
  - Here prostaglandin is lowering the Immunological Resistance.
  - *(Somatic or Corporeal) - Pathological Symptoms of Staphysagria.*
  - Colic after anger.
  - Severe pain following an abdominal procedure or operation? Iatrogenic.
  - Hypersensitivity.
  - Parts are very sensitive to touch. (so manipulations during laparoscopic examination results in to irritability and produces inflammation, regurgitation and colic and severe abdominal discomfort after Investigative procedures, hence this remedy is useful in – bad effects of surgery.
  - Urinary bladder is very sensitive with inflammation.
  - Inflammation of the ovaries.
  - Very Heavy Irregular Menses – comes late.
- **Thuja** (Arbor Vitae)
Miasm: Sycotic
  - *(Psycho) Psychological Symptoms of Thuja*
    - Highly emotional and sensitiveness
    - Thinking of herself as - made up of Glass – fragile.
    - Can not tolerate rough handling by spouse.
    - Sensation of being frail and fragile.
    - Low self esteem - feeling of worthlessness.
    - Feels unattractive—becomes cosmetic conscious.
    - Feels as if soul and body were separated.
    - Emotional sensitiveness
    - Music makes her to cry/ weep

- *(Somatic or Corporeal) Pathological Symptoms of Thuja.*
  - o Ill effects of vaccination (threat to immunity?)
  - o Vagina: very sensitive - vaginismus.
  - o Menses: scanty, retarded with pain in left iliac fossa and left ovary - worse on left side (adhesion)
  - o Profuse leucorrhoea.
  - o Abdomen: Distended - rumbling and colic.
  - o At every menstrual cycle
  - o Constipation with violent rectal pain. Dyschasia
- **Thiosinaminum** (Chemical Derived From the oil of Mustard seeds)
  - o It is a resolvent for dissolving scar tissues, tumours, glands, strictures, adhesions, Fibroids.
  - o It is very useful medicines for dissolving endometrial scar tissues.
- **Carcinosin** - the Nosode
  - o When well selected remedy fails to work on endometriosis
  - o Strong family history of carcinoma.
  - o Carcinoma of the uterus, mammary glands with pain and indurations.
  - o All the discharges are very offensive.
  - o Helps to build up the immunity in cancerous cachexia.
  - o Restoring back the hair after chemo-therapy
  - o When endometriosis turns to cancerous changes

19. ENDOMETRITIS

Endometritis refers to inflammation of the endometrial lining of uterus.

- **Causes**

  o Chlamydia
  o Gonococcal Endometritis
  o Salpingitis
  o Tubercular Endometritis

It can occur after

  o Child birth
  o Abortion – therapeutic, elective, spontaneous
  o IUCD
  o Any gynaecological procedure or surgery, which requires insertion of medical instruments.

Rubrics to select

- An inflammation of Endometrium

  o Apis, Ars, Bell, Canth, Lyco, Puls, Sabina, Secale Cor
  o Calendula, Haemm, Tiliea, Europaea.

- Female Genitalia / sex:

- Inflammation: Uterus
  o After abortion: Sabina, Tilia Europaea
  o After Haemorrhage: China, Millefolium
  o After Labour: Sabina, Sec.Cor
  o During Menses: Phosphorous
  o After surgery: Staphysagria

20. FIBROID

A benign smooth muscle tumour usually occurs in uterine muscle and tissue is known as fibroid.

Symptoms

- o Heavy menstrual bleeding
- o Prolonged Menstrual Period
- o Intermittent bleeding (bleeding between two periods)
- o Pelvic pressure or pain or discomfort
- o Urinary incontinence
- o Frequent urination or retention of urine
- o Constipation
- o Backache or leg cramps

Types

- Submoucosal – buldge into uterine cavity
- Subserosal – projects outside of uterine cavity
- Intramural – grows within the muscular uterine wall
- Pendunculated – hangs from a stalk or outside the uterus

Rubrics to select

- o Calc Carb
- o Calc Flour
- o Conium
- o Phosphorous
- o Thiosinaminum
- o Silicea
- o Arnica
- o Apis
- o Calc.Iod
- o Iodinum
- o Ledum
- o Tilia Europaea

21. GALACTORRHOEA (Hyper lactation)

Hyper lactation is the spontaneous flow the milk from the breasts; unrelated to childbirth or nursing. It is linked to elevated levels of prolactin.

Galactorrhoea may be associated with excessive breast stimulation; side effects of medicine or pituitary or hypothalamic disorder. This condition can be seen in men too.

Rubrics to select:

- Milk: Non Pregnant Woman with nodule of mamma
    - o Chimaphia Umbellata
    - o Lac Can
    - o Phytolecca-Q
    - o Thyroidinum

- Milk in Boys:

    - o Merc. Cor

- Milk at Puberty:

    - o Pulsatilla

22. HABITUAL ABORTION

It is the occurrence of repeated pregnancies that end in miscarriage of the foetus, usually before 20 weeks of gestation. There are three or more consecutive spontaneous abortions that occur at about the same stage of pregnancy. Habitual abortion usually occurs due to chromosomal abnormalities (usually chromosomal rearrangements) or other genetic causes.

- **Abortion 1ˢᵗ Trimester**

  - 1ˢᵗ month.
    - Apis Mellifica^{+++}
    - Caulophylum^{++}
    - Viburnum Opulus $^{++}$

  - Six weeks –One & half month
    - Ipeca
    - Sanguin
    - Spongia

  - Eight weeks-2ᵉᵈ month
    - Kali Carb
    - Cimicifuga
    - Sabina
    - Secal Cor

  - Twelve weeks -3ʳᵈ month
    - Apis Mel
    - Crocus Sat
    - Kreosotum
    - Trili. P
    - Eup. Perf, Merc Cor, Ustiligo
    - Kali carb
    - Sabina
    - Secalae. Cor.

- **Abortion 2nd Trimester**

  o Sixteen weeks - 4th Month

    o Apis
    o Caulophyllum
    o Eup.perf
    o Merc. cor

23. HYDATIDIFORM MOLE

It is a condition in which the tissue around the fertilised egg; called the chronic villi, develops as an abnormal cluster of cells and turns into grape like trophoblastic proliferation.
In other words, hydatidiform mole is a fleshy uterine tumour formed by degenerative or abortive development of an egg.

Cause
- Defect in ovum or follicle
- Uterine abnormalities
- Nutritional deficiencies

Rubrics to select
o Silicea
o Pulsatilla
o Nat. Carb
o Cimicifuga
o Belladonna
o China
o Merc. Cor
o Millefolium
o Sabina
o Helonias

24. HYDROSALPINX

In hydrosalpinx, there is an accumulation of serous fluid in the fallopian tube resulting in infertility.
Hydrosalpinx is a blocked, dilated, fluid filled fallopian tube, usually caused by a previous tubal infection or PID or STD.

Rubrics to select

- Female Genitalia/ sex:

    o Hydrosalpingitis:

    o **Gelsemium**

    o Calc Carb
    o Silicea
    o Apis Mel
    o Bryonia
    o Thiosinaminum

25. HYPERGLYCEMIA

Hyperglycemia, derived from a Greek, referring to excess sugar in the blood -

Hyper = too much

Glyc = root- meaning – sweet

Emia = suffix - meaning – of the blood

Causes

- Diabetes Mellitus
- Non – Diabetic
- Obesity
- Eating disorders like Bulimia Nervosa

- Diabetes:
  - Ars.Brom^{+++}
  - Bridelia Ferruginea^{+++}
  - Cocca^{+++}
  - Helleborus^{+++}
  - Morinda Lucida^{+++}
  - Natrum Sulph^{+++}
  - Opium^{++}
  - Phosphorous^{++}
  - Uranium Nitricum^{++}

- Non-Diabetic:
- Obesity:
  - Calc. Carb^{+++}
  - Graphitis^{+++}
  - Fuccus Vulgaris^{+++}
  - Phytolecca^{++}
  - Thyroidinum^{++}

- Eating disorders like Bulimia Nervosa

Rubric:

Appetite: Diminished:
  - Ginko biloba

26. HYPERTHYROIDISM (Hyper-thyroxineamia)

Hyperthyroidism is a clinical syndrome characterised by an excess of circulating free thyroxin (T4) or free triiodothyronine (T3) or sometimes both.

Cause
- Graves' disease
- Toxic thyroid adenoma
- Toxic Multi-nodular goitre

Signs and symptoms
- Hyperactivity
- Weight loss often accompanied by ravenous hunger
- Heat intolerance
- Fatigue and weakness
- Irritability, Apathy, Depression
- Polyuria—Increased frequency of Urination
- Sweating
- Palpitations
- Arrhythmias; especially Atrial Fibrillation
- Dyspnoea
- Loss of libido
- Nausea
- Vomiting
- Diarrhoea
- Neurological symptoms
- Tremors
- Chorea
- Myopathy
- Stroke

Rubric:
Ext. Throat: Swelling, Thyroid gland
Ext. Throat: Goitre
Pulsation: Goitre
Exophthalmic Goitre

Homeopathic Remedies:
- o Iodium
- o Kali iod
- o Flouric acid
- o Platina
- o Ars alb.
- o Thyroid
- o Conium
- o Thuja

27. HAEMORRHAGE

Haemorrhage is a medical term for bleeding, i.e. escape of blood to extra vascular space. Rapid, profuse haemorrhage causes shock and may prove fatal if the circulating volume can not be replaced in time. Slow, sustained bleeding may lead to anaemia. Arterial Bleeding is potentially more serious than blood lost from vein.

Rubric:
Female / Genitalia / Sex
    Haemorrhage = Metrorrhagia

Homeopathic Remedies:
Active:
- o Adrenaline
- o Belladonna
- o Calc Carb
- o Hamamelis
- o Phosphorous
- o Sanguinaria
- o Sabina
- o China
- o Ipeca
- o Millefolium
- o Trilium P
- o Strontium Carb

Passive:
- o Carb. Veg.
- o Erigeron Canadense
- o Kreosotum-Q
- o Trilium -P
- o Ustiligo
- o Sec.cor
- o Sepia

28. HIRSUITISM (Virilism)

Hirsuitism is defined as the excessive growth of thick, dark hair in locations where hair growth in women is minimal or absent like face, chest etc.

Hirsuitism in women means hair follicles are being over-stimulated by testosterone or other androgen hormones.

It can be **caused** by abnormally high androgen level observed at

- Puberty
- Masculinization
- Menopause
- Peri-menopause
- Ovarian tumour
- Adrenal hyperplasia
- Pituitary tumour

Rubric:

Face: Hair: Growth of hair: in women

- Chin
  - o Ignatia
  - o Olium J,

Upper lip:

- Cortica
- Hydros
- Natrum .Mur
- Oleum Jacoris
- Ignatia
- Thuja
- Testes
- Medorrhinum
- Natrum Mur
- Sepia,
- Thyrodinum

29. HYPOTHYROIDISM

It is a state of disease caused by insufficient production of thyroid hormone by the thyroid gland.

Cause:

Consumption of fluoride in excess, (e.g. tap water, sodas, bottled water). All drinks contain added water soluble fluorides.
Thyroid hormones are essential and "primary regulators" of the body metabolism.

Precautions:

Fluoride binds with iodine and prevents it from entering into thyroid. Iodine supplements may reverse the hypothyroidism.

Homeopathic Remedies:

- o Arg. nit
- o Calc. carb
- o Lycopodium
- o Thyroidinum

30. INCOMPETENT CERVIX
Weakened cervix which opens prematurely during pregnancy resulting into foetal loss.

Rubrics:

- Female genitalia/ sex:
- Swollen: Uterus
- Swollen : Cervix
- Indurations: Uterus: Cervix

Homeopathic Remedies:

- Aurum^{+++}
- Conium $^{+++}$
- Caulophyllum^{+++}
- Sepia^{+++}
- Iodium^{++}
- Platina^{++}
- Silicea^{++}

31. INCOMPLETE ABORTION

Abortion presented with lower abdominal cramping associated with vaginal bleeding. In this condition part of the foetus or placental material has retained within the uterus.

Rubric:

- Female/ Genitalia / Sex

- Contractions Uterus Os uteri

Homeopathic Remedies:

- Belladonna^{+++}
- Caulophyllum^{+++}
- Cimicifuga^{+++}
- Chammomilla^{+++}
- Erigeron Cand^{+++}
- Pulsatilla^{+++}
- Sec cor^{+++}
- Sepia^{+++}
- Sabina^{+++}
- Conium^{++}
- Gelsemium^{++}
- Vert. V.$^{++}$

32. MENORRHAGIA
Menorrhagia refers to heavy or prolonged menstrual flow.
Haemorrhage = Metrorrhagia
Homeopathic Remedies:
Active:

- o Adrenaline
- o Belladonna
- o Calc.Carb
- o Hamamelis
- o Phosphorous
- o Sanguinaria
- o Sabina
- o China
- o Ipeca
- o Millefolium
- o Trilium P
- o Strontium Carb

Passive:

- o Carb. Veg.
- o Erigeron
- o Kreosotum
- o Trilium-P
- o Ustiligo
- o Sec.cor
- o Sepia

33. METRORRHAGIA

Metrorrhagia involves menstrual spotting during middle of cycle, i.e. uterine bleeding at irregular intervals, particularly between the expected menstrual periods.

Causes: It occurs because of
- Hormonal imbalance
- Endometriosis
- Uterine fibroid
- Cancer (rarely)

Rubric:

Haemorrhage = Metrorrhagia

Homeopathic Remedies:

- **Active:**
  - Adrenaline
  - Belladonna
  - Calc.Carb
  - Ferrum Phos.
  - Hamamelis
  - Phosphorous
  - Sanguinaria
  - Sabina
  - China
  - Ipeca
  - Millefolium
  - Trilium P
  - Strontium Carb

- **Passive:**
  - Carb. Veg.
  - Erigeron
  - Kreosotum
  - Trilium-P
  - Ustiligo
  - Sec.cor
  - Sepia

34. MISCARRIAGE

A natural or spontaneous end of pregnancy at a stage where the embryo or the foetus is incapable of surviving generally defined at gestation of or prior to 20 weeks is known as miscarriage.

Spontaneous loss of embryo or foetus from uterus at gestation of 20 weeks or prior to it.

Homeopathic Remedies:

- o Bacillinum
- o Pulsatilla
- o Sepia
- o Syphillinum

Please refer first chapter Abortion for more detail. (page79)

35. MISSED ABORTION (Carnious mole)

A natural pre-mature expulsion of the products of conception like the embryo or non – viable foetus, from the uterus is known as missed abortion.

Rubrics:

- Female Genitalia/Sex: as if everything would escape
- Female Genitalia/Sex - Foetus - motions - palpitation from first movement of foetus
- Female Genitalia/Sex - Foetus motions with violent - vomiting;
- Female Genitalia/Sex - Movements - like a foetus
- Female Genitalia/Sex - Movement - of foetus
- Female Genitalia/Sex - Pain - labour pains - ascend with every pain; foetus seems to
- Female Genitalia/Sex - sensation as if uterus too small to pass foetus
- Generals - Faintness - pregnancy, during - motion of foetus; from slightest.

Homeopathic Remedies:

- o Apis Mel
- o Cantharis
- o Caulophyllum
- o Silicea
- o Sepia

36. MYOMA

It is a mesenchymal tumour.

- The leiomyoma; it is a common form of uterine fibroid.
- The rhabdomyoma: rarely occurs in muscle.
- Myoma is benign tumour of smooth muscle in the wall of uterus.
- A myoma of the uterus is often called Fibroid.

Homeopathic Remedies:

- o Calc. Carb^{+++}
- o Calc. Flour^{+++}
- o Lycopodium^{+++}
- o Phosphorous^{+++}
- o Silicea^{+++}
- o Terebinthina^{+++}
- o Apis^{++}
- o Conium^{++}
- o Kali Iod^{++}
- o Sec.Cor^{++}

37. OLIGOMENORRHOEA

Infrequent or very light menstruation in women at child bearing age is known as oligo-menorrhoea. Menstrual period occur at intervals of greater than 35 days, with only 4 to 9 periods in a year. It is very common to women at the beginning and end of their reproductive lives to miss or to have irregular periods.

Cause

- Imperfect co-ordination between the hypothalamus, the pituitary gland and ovaries.
- Emotional stress
- Chronic illness
- Excessive exercise
- Oestrogen secreting tumours
- Anabolic steroids
- Prolactinomas (Adenoma of the Anterior Pituitary)
- Thyrotoxicosis
- Grave's Disease

Homeopathic Remedies:

- o Janosia Asoca-Q
- o Pulsatilla-Q
- o Caulophyllum-Q
- o Sepia-Q
- o Ammonium Carb
- o Belladonna^{+++}
- o Caulophyllum^{+++}
- o Conium^{+++}
- o Cyclamen^{+++}
- o Ipeca^{++}
- o Graphitis^{++}
- o Lachesis^{++}
- o Ovarium^{++}
- o Pulsatilla^{++}
- o Veratrum Alb^{++}

38. ORGASMIC DISORDERS (Sexual Arousal Disorder)

In orgasmic disorders, there is a persistent or recurrent failure to achieve and maintain the lubrication-swelling response of sexual excitement and compilation of sexual activity.

Causes:

- Psychological and Acquired Causes
  - Marital Discord-Fear-Abuse
  - Depression
  - Lack of Knowledge of Genitalia functions
  - Feelings of Sin and Guilt
- Physical Causes
  - Localised Disease-Endometriosis, Cystitis, Vaginitis, Salpingitis
  - Systemic Disease-Hypo Thyroidism, Diabetes, Hypertension
  - CNS Diseases: Multiple sclerosis, Muscular Dystrophy
  - Iatrogenic=caused by medication like oral contraceptive, anti-hypertensive, anti-depressant, tranquilisers
  - Smoking and Alcohol, Recreational drugs.
  - Surgery-like Hysterectomy, Mastectomy
  - Aging: Atrophy of the vaginal mucosa leading to dryness and difficulty in developing enough vaso congestion.

Rubrics to select:

Female Genitalia /Sex
  - Aversion to sex
  - Inflammation - Ovaries - sexual excesses; from
  - Inflammation - Uterus - sexual excesses, after
  - Leucorrhoea - constant, chronic sexual desire; with increased
  - Leucorrhoea - sexual excitement, from
  - Lochia - sexual desire; with increased
  - Menses - absent - sexual desire
  - Menses - pale - sexual desire; with loss of
  - Menses - scanty - sexual desire lost
  - Pain - Ovaries - sexual desire, during
  - Sexual Desire - diminished - ovulation; during - accompanied by – weakness

Homeopathic Remedies:

- Argentum Nitricum^{+++}
- Berberis Vulgaris^{+++}
- Bromium^{+++}
- Calcarea Carb^{+++}
- Platina^{+++}
- Natrum Mur^{+++}
- Arsenicum Album^{++}
- Caladium^{++}
- Lilium Tig^{++}
- Murex^{++}
- **Mangifera Indica-Q**$^{++}$
- Opium^{++}
- Palladium^{++}

39. OVARIAN CYST

Ovarian cyst refers to the fluid filled sac inside the ovary.

The term cyst refers to a fluid filled structure. Usually an ovarian cyst is functional and occurs as a normal process of ovulation.

When the mature cyst does not rupture and grows bigger in size, then it turns into ovarian cyst.

Symptoms

- Abdominal pain
- Constant dull, aching, pelvic pain
- Dysparunia
- Shifting pain
- Dyschasia means Pain during passing stool.
- DUB (Dysfunctional Uterine Bleeding)
- Amenorrhoea
- Abdominal bloating

Homeopathic Remedy:

- General
  - Apis
  - Baptisia
  - Bovista
  - Bufo Rana
  - Cantharis
  - Colocynth
  - Iodium
  - Platina
  - Thuja
- Rt. Sided Ovarian Cyst
  - Apis Mel
  - Lycopodium
  - Rhus Tox
- Lt. Sided Ovarian Cyst
  - Argentum Nit
  - Lachesis
  - Podophyllum

40. OVULATORY FAILURE (Anovulation)

Anovulation is a condition in which the ovary does not release a matured follicle each month as a part of woman's normal cycle in her reproductive years. It refers to absence of ovulation or failure to ovulate

Factors responsible for Anovulation:

- Stress, new environment
- Chronic mental illness, such as depression
- Chronic physical illness, such as inflammatory bowel disease, poorly controlled diabetes, tuberculosis, or anaemia
- Under nutrition, specific nutrient deficiencies, inadequate body fat
- Prolonged or continuous physical exertion
- Various pharmaceutical (especially phenothiazines) and recreational drugs
- Hormone imbalances, such as prolactin or testosterone excess (e.g., polycystic ovary syndrome), hyper or hypothyroidism, adrenal insufficiency or Cushing's syndrome.
- Pituitary or ovarian failure.
- Taking birth control pills:

Rubrics to select:

Abdomen - Heaviness - ovulation; during

Abdomen- Pain - ovulation; during

Abdomen - Pain - Hypogastrium - ovulation; during

Abdomen - Pain - cutting - ovulation; during

Rubrics...

Female Genitalia/ Sex

Ovulation; during

Pain - Ovaries - ovulation, at

Pain- cutting - ovulation; during

Pain- cutting - Ovaries - right - ovulation; during

Sexual Desire - diminished - ovulation; during

Sexual desire- diminished - ovulation; during accompanied by - weakness

Back Pain - aching - ovulation; during

Generals-Weakness- accompanied by sexual desire; diminished - ovulation; during

Homeopathic Remedies:

- o Apis
- o Conium
- o Folliculinum
- o Iodium
- o Pulsatilla

41. PELVIC INFLAMMATORY DISEASE (PID)

It is a general term for infection of the female uterus, fallopian tube and/or ovaries, as it progresses to scar formation with adhesions to nearby tissues and organs.

It is an infection of pelvic organs; causes severe illness, fever and extreme pain.

Causes

- STD
- Past abortions
- Viral
- Fungal / Parasitic / Bacterial
- Mechanical—IUCD
- Haematogenous

Homeopathic Remedies:

- Apis^{+++}
- Belladonna^{+++}
- Calc Carb^{+++}
- Hepar Sulph^{+++}
- Bryonia^{++}
- Merc Cor^{++}
- Palladium^{++}
- Silicea^{++}

42. PREMENSTRUAL SYNDROME (PMS)

Premenstrual syndrome (PMS) is a group of symptoms linked to the menstrual cycle. It involves a variety of physical, mental and behavioural symptoms linked to menstruation. It usually occurs between ages of 40-50. PMS is shorter, usually milder and involves more physical symptoms.

Symptoms

- o Anxiety, Apprehension, Depression, Mood Swing
- o Acne, Multiple boils on face
- o Appetite: change in food craving
- o Breast swelling and tenderness
- o Difficulty in concentrating
- o Constipation / Diarrhoea
- o Depression
- o Headache
- o Sleeplessness
- o Emotional disturbances
- o Swelling: Breasts / Legs

Pre menstrual Dysphoric Disorder

Is characterised by symptoms like -

- • Mood swing
- • Depression
- • Anxiety and Irritability that occur prior to period=PMT
- • Physical symptoms such as bloating and cramping.

Homeopathic Remedies:

- o Graphitis^{+++}
- o Lachesis^{+++}
- o Pulsatilla^{+++}
- o Sec Cor^{+++}
- o Sepia^{+++}
- o Calc. Carb^{++}
- o Nat.Mur. $^{++}$

43. UTERINE POLYP

It is a benign growth within the uterine cavity, originating from endometrium that takes up space within the uterine cavity. The uterine or endometrial polyp consists of area of uterus where endometrium becomes overgrown and forms a polyp. A polyp is an abnormal overgrowth of tissue (tumour) projecting from a mucus membrane. If it is attached to the surface by a narrow elongated stalk, it is called pedunculated. If no stalk is present, it is called sessile.

Polyps are commonly found in the colon, stomach, nose, urinary bladder and uterus.

They may also occur elsewhere in the body where mucus membrane exists like cervix and small intestine.

Homeopathic Remedies:

- o Belladonna^{+++}
- o Calc.Carb $^{+++}$
- o Phosphorous^{+++}
- o Teucrum marum $^{+++}$
- o Thuja^{+++}
- o Bryonia^{++}
- o Bufo^{++}
- o Conium^{++}
- o Calc. Flour^{++}
- o Lycopodium^{+++}
- o Platina^{++}
- o Sepia^{++}
- o Silicea^{++}

44. RETROVERTED UTERUS

Anatomically the position of the Uterus is Ante-verted and Ante-flexed, but the condition where Uterus that is tilted backwards instead of forward, is called as "Retroverted" Uterus.

Causes

- Congenital
- Acquired
  - Pelvic surgery
  - Pelvic adhesions
  - Endometriosis
  - PID
  - Labour / Childbirth
  - Any condition that causes an increase in the intra abdominal pressure.

Rubric:

Displacement of Uterus

Homeopathic Remedies:

- Aesculus[+++]
- Belladonna[+++]
- Calc.Carb[+++]
- Lil.Tig[+++]
- Platina[+++]
- Natrum.Mur[+++]
- Sepia[+++]
- Staphysagria[+++]
- Abies Canadensis[++]
- Caulophyllum[++]
- Cimicifuga[++]
- Lachesis[++]
- Thuja[++]

45. SALPINGITIS

Salpingitis is the inflammation of one or both fallopian tubes caused by bacterial, viral or fungal or mechanical cause.

The inflammation induces the secretion of serous fluid or even pus to collect inside the fallopian tube.

Most common bacteria responsible for Salpingitis are:

- Chlamydia
- Gonococcal-Neiserria Gonorrhoeae
- Mycoplasma
- Staphylococcal
- Viral: Mumps

Causes: Factors inviting Infection:

- Unprotected Sexual Intercourse
- Miscarriage
- Abortion/ MTP
- Child Birth
- Intra Uterine Contraceptive Device-IUCD
- Secondary Metastasis from Appendix

Homeopathic Remedies:

- o Arsenicum Album
- o Apis Mel
- o Baptisia
- o Belladonna
- o Parotidinum
- o Sepia

46. SEPTATE UTERUS

In this condition fibrous septum separates the uterine cavity into two compartments.

It is due to of resorption of the final fibrous septum between the Muller ducts.

Septate uterus consists of a single uterus divided by a large fibrous midline septum – because of mullerian duct abnormality.

Two mullerian ducts are fusing together to form a single uterus.

Types:

- Complete
- Sub-septate

o No any specific Homeopathic Remedies, as it is a gross anatomical abnormality.

47. STILL BIRTH (IUFD - Intra Uterine Foetal Death)

A still birth is defined as the death of the foetus at anytime after the 20th week of gestation.

Causes:

- Bacterial infection, Viral Infection-TORCH
- Genetic defect / Birth defect
- Chromosomal abnormalities
- Growth retardation
- Maternal risk factors
- illness like diabetes/ high blood pressure
- consumption of Tobacco, Nicotine, Alcohol
- prolonged medication

Homeopathic Remedies:

Refer Abortion page 79

48. URINARY TRACT INFECTION (UTI)

Symptoms:

- Strong and persistent urge to urinate
- Nocturia – Night frequency
- Urethritis – discomfort and pain at urethral meatus
- Dysuria – burning sensation throughout the urethra while urination
- Cystis – pain in the middle of supra pubic region
- Haematuria – presence of blood / pus in the urine
- Fever with rigors
- Emesis – vomiting
- Fever with Rigors

Homeopathic Treatment:

- o Apis
- o Berberis Vulg.
- o Cantharis
- o Equisitum
- o Sarsaparilla
- o Staphysagria
- o Terebenthina Oleum

Useful Mother Tinctures:

- o Berberis Vulgaris-Q
- o Calendula-Q
- o Staphysagria-Q

49. VAGINISMUS

Vaginismus is involuntary vaginal tightness causing discomfort, burning pain, penetration problems or complete inability of intercourse, consequently, vaginal penetration during sex is difficult or impossible.

Types

1. Primary:
- Usually occurs in teenagers and in early 20 s.
- Attempt to use Tampons.
- Having forced penetrative Sex.
- Undergoing Gynaecological Examination or Smear Test
- Pre-fixed Ideas, Lack of Knowledge, Illiteracy.
- Fear of pain of breaking Hymen at first attempt of sexual act.
- Sexual abuse, Rape, Incest

2. Secondary
- Infection like Candidiasis, Moniliasis, Giardiasis etc
- Injury- Trauma, Post Surgical stricture.
- Post Episiotomy pain

Causes:

Psychological:
- It results from woman `s Sub-conscious desire to avoid sex.
- Post painful sexual experience
- Fear Of Guilt, becoming pregnant, Sinful act, Religious myths.
- Fear of Domination from partner.
- Fear of loss of self control.

Physical:
- Pelvic Infection
- Scar and Contracture resulting due to Injury after surgery or at Child birth, Episiotomy repair, forceps, vacuum delivery etc.
- Constant Irritation due to IUCD, Douches, Tampons,
- Irritation from Latex in Condom and Spermicides.

Homeopathic Remedies:

- Argentum Nitricum^{+++}
- Cactus^{+++}
- Nat. Mur^{+++}
- Sepia^{+++}
- Belladonna^{++}
- Berberis Vulgaris^{++}
- Cantharis^{++}
- Caulophyllum^{++}
- Cimicifuga^{++}

50. VAGINITIS

Inflammation of vaginal mucosa often associated with an irritation or infection of the vulva leading to vulvo-vaginitis.

Causes:

1. Infection: Infection caused by Bacteria, Parasites, Yeasts
   - Candidia Albicantis
   - Trichomonas Vaginalis
   - Giardiasis
   - Gardnerella
   - Enterobius Vermicularis
   - Gonorrhoeal
   - Chlamydia
   - Mycoplasma
   - Herpes etc.
2. Hormonal Vaginitis:
   - Puberty
   - Post partum
   - Post menopausal
3. Irritation: due to various Allergies
4. Foreign Bodies: Retained Tampons

Homeopathic Remedies:

- Aconite^{+++}
- Belladonna^{+++}
- Hamamelis $^{+++}$
- Merc.Sol^{+++}
- Skukoom^{+++}
- Sepia^{+++}
- Alumina^{++}
- Caulophyllum^{++}
- Hypericum^{++}
- Nitric Acid^{++}
- Rhus Tox^{++}
- Sepia^{++}

51. WARTS (Condylomata)

Condyloma comes a from Greek word

Condylomata acuminate = Genital warts

Condylomata lata = a white lesion associated with syphilis

- Condylomata Acuminate

Small, pointed Papilloma of viral origin usually occurs on the skin or mucus surface of the external genitalia or peri anal region.

Other terms for Condylomata acuminate

- Ano-genital venereal warts
- Genital warts
- Veneral warts
- Verruca accuminata

Cause:

- Human Papilloma Virus (HPV)
- Multiple sexual partners
- Unknown partners
- Early onset of sexual activities
- Tobacco
- Nutritional status
- Hormonal causes
- Age
- Stress
- Concurrent viral infections, such as Influenza, HIV,Herpes etc.

Site:

- Vulva
- Urethra
- Vagina
- Cervix and
- Peri anal regions

Homeopathic Remedies:

- Cannaberis^{+++}
- Hepar Sulph^{+++}
- Natrum Sulph^{+++}
- Nitric Acid^{+++}
- Sepia^{+++}
- Thuja^{+++}
- Anacardium Occidentalis^{++}
- Lycopodium^{++}
- Medorrhinum^{++}
- Merc.Sol. $^{++}$
- Phosph.Acid^{++}
- Sepia^{+++}
- Staphysagria^{++}

MIASMATIC EVALUATION OF SEXUAL SYMPTOMS

PSORIC SEXUAL SYMPTOMS
- All functional and psychological menstrual disorders
- DUB=Dysfunctional Uterine Bleeding
- Leucorrhoea
- Psoric discharge are always *Bland*
- Because of prolonged sufferings of the exhaustive disease - weakness of sexual organs
- Excessive and very high sexual desire
- Full moon and New moon aggravation.

SYPHILITIC SEXUAL SYMPTOMS
- Inability to perform- Erectile Dysfunction
- Decreased Sexual Desire-Low Libido
- All cancers – Penis, Uterus
- Breast Involvement with offensive discharge P/V
- Offensive odour – Vagina (Vaginitis)
- Hypersensitive Vagina—Pain
- Fainting after menses
- Depression + Fear – Menses
- Recurrent abortions
- Azospermia in Male

SYCOTIC SEXUAL SYMPTOMS
- Mind always concentrated on sex organs and sexual Fancies
- Acrid Leucorrhoea – Smells like fish or Putrid odour
- Sterility + Infertility
- Hyper Prolactinaemia
- Various Menstrual Disorders-Meno, Metro and Poly menorrhoea
- Itching Pudenda – Pruritus Vulvae – Mastodynia (Painful Breast)
- Menses – Offensive smell--Smells like Fish Brine
- Stains of menses – difficult to wash off
- Mental weakness during Leucorrhoea

TUBERCULAR SEXUAL SYMPTOMS

- Spermatorrhoea
- Masturbation– Loss of all enthusiasm, depression, weakness of memory
- Emission of semen during : Defecation or Micturition
- Uterine Ovarian and Allied Complications.
- Profound Weakness
- Profound Bright red bleeding P/V – (DUB)
- Continues or persist for a long time and reoccurs again Diarrhoea, Fever, Visual Auditory Hallucination, Anorexia, Nausea, Vomiting during menses

FACTORS AFFECTING FERTILITY

The number of cases of infertility is increasing rapidly. It has been found that 8-12% males of all the male infertility cases reported are functionally sterile, i.e. their sperm count per millilitre of semen is less than 20 million. Furthermore, it has been reported that about 40% of all infertility cases are due to male factors. The factors affecting infertility are listed as follows -

- **Effect of Tobacco:** (smoking, chewing, brushing, snuffing)

Sperm counts of the tobacco smokers are on average 13—17 % lower than non-smokers. The toxic chemicals like nicotine in the smoke are responsible for lowering sperm count. As a consequence of abnormal mutagenic activity, male smokers have an increase in sperm abnormalities.

A high number of abnormal sperm heads is associated with decreased their acrosomal activities and hence decreased fertilisation. An elevated level of abnormal sperm is an indication of the decreased mutagenic potency in spermatogenesis.

Bad effects of tobacco: Lobelia –Q is a Remedy of Choice.

- It acts as a vaso-motor stimulant.
- Increases the activity of all vegetative process, by spending its force upon the Pneumo- gastric nerve which produces the depressed, relaxed condition with oppression of chest and Epigastrium.
- It also suppresses the discharges.
- Bad effect of Drunkenness.
- Profuse Salivation with good appetite.
- Dyspnoea from constriction of chest

Some more Homeopathic Remedies to counter the bad effects of Tobacco

- o Tabacum—Q
- o Strychninum
- o Ignatia
- o Pulsatilla
- o Spigelia

- **PESTICIDES: CHEMICALS**

It has been reported by Dr. Baranski (Institute of Occupational Medicine, Copenhagen, Denmark) that chemicals like those in textile dyes, dry-cleaning chemicals, lead, mercury, cadmium etc. cause ill-effects on sperms. Such chemicals have been shown to reduce sperm numbers and damage the quality of sperms, and seminiferous tubules (site of sperm production)

The highest number of cases of infertility-related, low-sperm counts were found in agricultural jobs. Also, a significant number of cases have been found in people involved with doing damp proofing or termite treatment, as the chemicals used contain chlordane. Furthermore, people living in houses given the above mentioned treatments have also been found to have low-sperm count.

The pesticide "Chlorpyrifos" is responsible to cause increase in auto-immune antibodies in people exposed to the pesticide.

- **WATER**

Factors like hyper-chlorinated water and fluoride content of water are also known to affect the morphological aspects of sperm and lower their numbers.

- **EXPOSURE TO SOLVENTS: HIGH RISK:**
  o Perchlorethylene (used in laundry for dry cleaning)
  o Trichloroethylene (used in laundry for dry cleaning)
  o Paint Thinners
  o Paint Strippers.
  o Ziram
  o Thiram
  o Dithane-M 45
  o Chlorpyrifos (responsible for increase in auto-immune antibodies in exposed workers)

Risk of infertility increases in female exposure to textile dyes, dry cleaning chemicals, noise, lead, mercury and cadmium. Furthermore, workers exposed to certain types of bulk drugs, paints, chemicals, brass polishing, medicines, cosmetics etc experience certain types of abnormalities in their fertility profile, depending on time and severity of exposure.

Cases of premature deliveries, small birth weight and still birth are higher in chemically exposed women and those working in a plastic or synthetics industries, textile industries where chemicals, dyes, plastic, formaldehydes. Similar cases are seen in women whose husbands work with these types of agents.

Furthermore, men living in industrial cities have shown 8-10 times lower sperm counts compared to those living in non-industrial areas, thus indicating a correlation between chemical exposure and low sperm counts.

• CARBON EXHAUST EMITTED BY VEHICLES

Vehicle exhausts containing carbon and Benzo(a)Pyrene (BaP) and lead, when inhaled significantly reduce and seriously affect the fertility parameters in male and female. Furthermore, these also cause reduction in ovarian weight and marked reduction in ovarian follicles in females.

• COFFEE:

Coffee drinking has also been associated with infertility. Data suggests that consumption of 1 cup coffee per day increases 55% higher risk of not conceiving.

2-3 cups of coffee per day increases the risk by 100% and more than 3 cups increases the risk by 176%. Furthermore, consumption of more than 3 cups of coffee per day before and after pregnancy increases the risk of miscarriage.

• ALCOHOL AND RECREATIONAL DRUGS:

Intoxicating effects of alcohol reduces the chances of conception by 50% in males by affecting gametogenesis in humans.

Recreational Drugs

o Recreational drugs cause blockage of nervous pathways in to the hypothalamus.

o Hypothalamus controls the parasympathetic nervous system.

o It is an important reflex centre for emotional expression and sexual function. With the recreational drugs when this pathway gets blocked, then it reflects on sexual functions by suppressions of most if not all the hormones.

- Opium:

In certain parts of India, opium consumption is customary to welcome guests. More cases of infertility (esp, impotent males and males with abnormal sperm morphology) have been reported from such areas.

- Cocaine:

Cocaine binds on to the sperm and finds its way in to the egg during the process of fertilisation, which either results in to abnormal sperm morphology or abnormal development of foetus.

- Marijuana:

Marijuana has anovulatory effects in females by suppressing the nervous pathways in to the hypothalamus.

• ANAESTHESIA:

The anaesthetist nurses and staff have a higher risk of birth-defect in their children because of constant exposure and inhalation of volatile anaesthetic agents.

Exposure to anaesthesia is responsible for causing sperm damage and it is also linked with increases the risk of sperm abnormalities by 50% compared to that in normal male.

MEDICAL FERTILITY TREATMENT:

1. Clomiphene
2. Human Chorionic Gonadotrophin (HCG)
3. Human Menopausal Gonadotrophin (HMG)
4. Anabolic Steroids

It has been said that "anything in excess is poison" same way...

Administration of FSH (Follicle Stimulating Hormone) is the most common treatment of infertility. This results in persistent stimulation of ovaries by gonadotrophin or its analogues, thus having direct effects on raised oestrogen level in serum.

1. **CLOMIPHENE CITRATE** is an oestrogen derivative and its side-effects are as follows.
   - Vaso-motor Flushes
   - Abdominal Distension
   - Breast Tenderness
   - Nausea
   - Visual Disturbances
   - Headache
   - Multiple pregnancies - Primarily Twins.
   - Ovarian Hyper stimulations resulting in to PCOD and at later stage
     (Stein-Lewanthal syndrome)

2. **HUMAN CHORIONIC GONADOTROPHIN (HCG)**
   Side-effects
   - Headache.
   - Irritability
   - Restlessness
   - Depression
   - Fatigue
   - Oedema
   - Precocious Puberty
   - Sensitivity Reactions

3. HUMAN MENOPAUSAL GONADOTROPHIN (HMG)
- Sensitivity Reaction
- Ovarian Hyper stimulation with Enlargement or Rupture of Cyst
- Multiple Pregnancies.

4. ANABOLIC STEROIDS
- Increased Acne
- Musculo Tendinous sensitivity
- Gynaecomastia
- Azospermia
- Liver dysfunction
- Alopecia
- Hirsuitism---Hoarse Voice—Enlarged Clitoris
- Atrophy of Vaginal Mucosa

5. Gn-RH ANALOGUE
- Vomiting
- Headache
- Seizures
- Syncope
- Other CNS –Reaction.
- Peripheral Neuropathy.
- Metallic taste
- Dark Urine

Ovarian Hyper stimulation Syndrome results due to -
- Significant side effects
- Male and Female Factors must be adequately evaluated.

The major risk of HMG therapy is the ovarian hyper-stimulation syndrome. It can be life threatening with massive enlarged ovaries. The shift of an intra-vascular fluid volume in to the peritoneal space results in
- Hypovolaemia
- Oliguria
- Haemoconcentration
- Massive Ascitis

REPERTORY OF OBSTACLES TO FERTILITY

1. ILL-EFFECTS OF TOBBACCO
- o Lobelia
- o Tabacum
- o Strychninum
- o Ignatia
- o Nux vomica
- o Pulsatilla
- o Staphysagria
- o Spigelia

2. ILL-EFFECTS OF PESTICIDES
- o Rhus tox
- o Sepia
- o Ferrum met
- o Cantharis
- o Nat. Sulph
- o Ars.alb
- o Nux. Vom

3. ILL-EFFECTS OF EXHAUST (CARBONS)
- o Graphitis
- o Carbo veg
- o Carbolic acid

4. ILL-EFFECTS OF COFFEE
- o Coffeea cruda
- o Chammomila
- o Ignatia
- o Nux vom
- o Causticum

5. ILL-EFFECTS OF CHEMICALS
- o Carbolic acid
- o Benzoic acid
- o Sulphuric acid
- o Nitric acid
- o Flouric acid

6. ILL-EFFECTS OF COCCAINE
- o Coffea
- o Belladonna
- o Lechesis
- o Chammomila
- o Nux vom
- ' o Opium
- o Cannabis sativa

7. ILL-EFFECTS OF CHEMICAL IN DRINKING WATER
- o Cocculus
- o Arsenic
- o Croton tig
- o Pulsatilla
- o Flouric acid

8. ILL-EFFECTS OF ANAESTHESA
- o Abrotinum

9. ILL-EFFECTS OF ALCOHOL
- o Arsenic
- o Lachesis
- o Nux vom
- o Opium
- o Ran. Bulb
- o Sulphur
- o Sulphuric acid
- o Lycopodium
- o Coffea

10. ILL-EFFECTS OF MARIJUANA

o Cannabis sativa
o Strychnine
o Thiosinaminum

All these factors usually play very important role on fertility. These factors were referred to as noxious or morbiphic agents by Dr. Hahnemman, the father of Homeopathy. Almost everybody would come in direct or indirect contact with these; however the time-span of exposure and the severity of exposure play a crucial role in determining the long-term effects.

Some 200 years ago, pollutions, stress, tension were not much prevalent but it was his foresightedness and he gave an indication of the effects of these in his early days of research, which we are experiencing in our routine practice, now a days.

So, Homeopathic treatment is safe, secure, without side-effects, Sweet in taste and Non-invasive, which restores the sick to health.

References:

1. Banerjea, S. K.; 1994 Miasmatic Diagnosis, 1st Edition, B.Jain Publishers
2. Chatterjee, C. C, (1985), *Human Physiology*, II volume,
3. Dr. Jean Ginsburg, Male Infertility and Chemicals in Drinking water, London Royal Free Hospital Lancet, January,22.
4. K. Das, (1957), Clinical Methods in Surgery, 8th edition, Calcutta, the City Book Co.
5. Kristensen, P & Eilertsen, E.; (1995), Car Exhaust decreases Fertility, Envirnomental Health Perspectives, 103, pp: 588-590
6. Merk Manual—16th Edition
7. Merrian-Webster's dictionary [Online], http://www.merriam-webster.com/, (Accessed on 11 June 2009)
8. Oscar E. Boericke W. Boericke, (1927), *Homeopathic Materia Medica*, 9th edition, Kessinger Publishing Co.
9. Sinclair, W. & Pressinger, R.; (1993), *Risk from Medical Fertility Treatment*, Lancet, pp 987
10. Smith, C.; (1983), *Marijuana stops ovulation*, Science,March25,1983
11. Strokum, H, (1983), *Pesticides suspected of causing infertility*, American Journal of Industrial Medicine, 24, pp: 587:592